330 - 7020

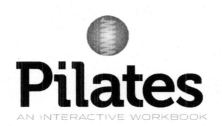

Pilates
AN INTERACTIVE WORKBOOK

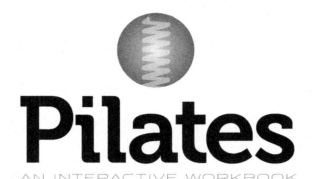

Pilates

AN INTERACTIVE WORKBOOK

If you're going to do it, do it right.

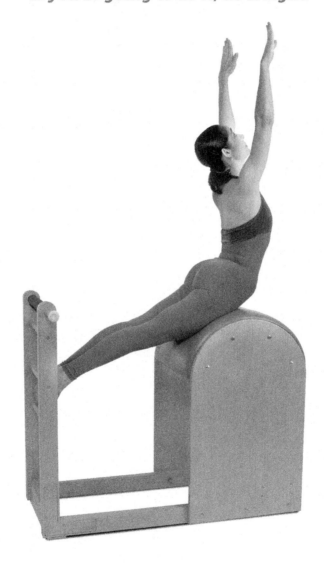

Christina Maria Gadar

2nd Generation Certified Pilates Instructor

Copyright © 2013 by Christina Maria Gadar

All rights reserved. The reproduction or utilization of this work in any form or by any electronic, mechanical, or other means, now known or hereafter invented, including xerography, photocopying, and recording, and in any information storage and retrieval system, is forbidden without the written permission of the copyright holder.

Gadar, Christina Maria.
Pilates an interactive workbook: if you're going to do it, do it right. / Christina Maria Gadar
ISBN-13: 978-0-6156-9795-6
ISBN-10: 0-6156-9795-X

Design: Max Kelly, Ulises Piedra
Photography (interior): Max Kelly Design
Photography (front and back cover): Blonde Cow Photography
Model: Christina Maria Gadar
Pilates Apparatus: Gratz Industries

This workbook is for educational purposes only and is not intended to replace learning Pilates from a certified Pilates instructor. Gadar Inc. d/b/a Gadar Pilates disclaims any and all liability for any adverse effects arising from the use or application of the information shown in this book.

To order more copies of *Pilates An Interactive Workbook*, visit:
www.pilatespersonaltraining.com

Dedication

I dedicate this book to my grandmother Haydée de Carvalho, the true writer in my family, who in addition to many other things, taught me the value of books and the value of doing things right.

I also dedicate this book to my Pilates mentor Romana Kryzanowska, who taught me the importance of doing everything with music in my soul, and to my ballet coach Fernando Bujones, who taught me at a very young age to live my life with sincerity, integrity and class. Both have made me the Pilates teacher I am today.

Acknowledgements

First and foremost, I must thank my Pilates mentor, Romana Kryzanowska. After Joseph Pilates died, it was Romana, along with Clara Pilates, who kept the studio running. Thanks to Romana, the Pilates Method as Joseph Pilates taught it has lived on. As a second generation Pilates instructor, I strive to teach Pilates in its purest form, as Joseph Pilates taught it to Romana, and as she taught it to me. Everything I do in the Pilates community is done with Romana in mind. Every article I write, every interview I do, every Pilates workout I film, and now this book, is done to educate people about the importance of preserving the integrity of Joseph Pilates' original vision of physical and mental conditioning.

I would also like to express my gratitude to all my Pilates teachers, who deepen my love for what I do each and every time I study with them. I have always learned the most from private Pilates lessons. There is no replacement for a teacher's personalized cue words, touch and energy. A sincere thank you goes to Sari Mejia Santo, Juanita Lopez, Cynthia Lochard, Roxane Richards-Huang, Anthony Rabara, Jerome Weinberg, Cynthia Shipley, Lori Coleman-Brown, Janice Dulak and Moses Urbano for their invaluable private Pilates instruction.

Grandmaster teachers Sari Mejia Santo and Juanita Lopez generously gave up their time to talk to me about my ideas for this book, as did master teachers Roxane Richards-Huang and Daria Pace. I hope I have found the right balance in producing a book that encourages dedicated Pilates students to practice safely at home and efficiently in the studio. **Please remember that this book is meant only for those who are already students of a certified Pilates instructor. Pilates *cannot* be learned from a book or a video–*only* from a teacher.**

This book would not exist without the expertise of Max Kelly Design. Max has that perfect combination of computer savvy and love of all things artistic. After creating my website, Max began Pilates training with me. When it came time to shoot the photos for this book, he was able to draw from his knowledge of Pilates to get the best shots. In various test photo shoots and a final photo shoot that lasted more than five hours, he shot over 2000 photographs with patience and precision. He was also able to take the book layout that was in my mind and put it to paper. Thank you, Max Kelly Design, you made my dream of contributing something meaningful to the Pilates community, a reality.

Thank you to Kollene and Mattias Carlsson of Blonde Cow Photography for the photos on the front and back cover. In addition to shooting all the photographs for my website, they photograph my family each year and have become wonderful friends.

The reformer apparatus, mat and magic circle featured in the photos are all from Gratz Industries based in Long Island, New York. Gratz Industries produces quality Pilates equipment that lasts a lifetime. Based on the original designs from Joseph Pilates, Gratz equipment, in combination with the instruction of a certified Pilates instructor, will change your body.

A special thank you goes to my students, who asked for this book, generously advised me on it, and waited for it with anxious anticipation. As an owner of a Pilates studio in a town with a distinct peak resident season, I was presented with the challenge of helping my students continue their Pilates training for the five or so months they go out of town each year. Many of my students have second homes in places without Pilates studios nearby. Even my students who live in town year round expressed the desire for a guide for their home-based workouts. I hope this workbook will help motivated Pilates students maintain consistency in their home-based workouts and keep them progressing in their Pilates lessons in the studio. An extra thank you goes to Judith Rock, my Pilates student since 2004, who generously took time away from her own writing to edit parts of this book.

Finally, I must thank my family for their huge support in all my endeavors. I thank my mother Mariluci Toloza, for always encouraging me to strive for excellence, and my sister Denise, for her helpful words of inspiration. I offer an extra special thank you to my incredibly supportive husband Filipp, and my two amazing children Marcelo and Taís Haydée, who understand that all good things take time, and have been wonderful about giving me time to make this book.

Contents

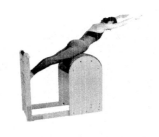

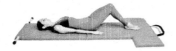
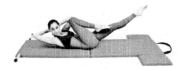
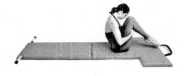
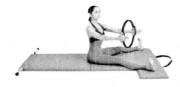

How To Use This Workbook

No Pilates book can reveal the depth of practice necessary to achieve an understanding of the Method's true essence. The only way to truly learn Pilates is to feel it in your own body *with the guidance of a certified Pilates instructor.* But once you have an instructor, practicing Pilates at home on your own is also an important element in taking ownership of your workout and making the most of the time and money you invest in your lessons. This book presents a general outline of many of the exercises you will encounter in your Pilates lessons, and since Pilates exercises need to be personalized and adapted on a continual basis, this workbook provides a place to record those modifications.

It is important to remember that you *never* perform any exercise on your own unless you have already practiced it in the studio with your instructor. Each series of workouts is in a specific order represented at the beginning of each chapter. For more details on a specific exercise, refer to the corresponding page number provided with the photo. If you get to an exercise that you need to omit, go to the next exercise in that series. For example, if you are practicing some of the basic seven mat exercises, but are not yet practicing the double leg stretch (exercise six) with your instructor, skip it and go to the spine stretch forward (exercise seven).

If you have enough space to put a bath towel on the floor, you have enough room to practice your matwork. In addition to the basic and intermediate level matwork, this workbook includes other useful exercises that can be performed at home. For example, you can use a magic circle to vary your matwork routine. You can also perform the standing weights series, magic circle exercises and ending wall series. Whether or not you have the magic circle and hand weights is not as important as the resistance you *create* as you perform the exercises. And all you need to perform the wall series is a wall.

The basic and intermediate reformer exercises are included in the workbook because they, with the matwork, are the heart and soul of the Pilates Method. Even if you don't have a reformer apparatus at home, reviewing the reformer exercises will help you prepare for your lessons with your instructor. You will spend less time during your lesson trying to remember how to set up the apparatus and do the exercise, and will have more time to concentrate on the intricacies of the movements.

This workbook has step-by-step photographs of all the exercises described, to help you connect the name of the exercise to its movement. In addition to photographs, every exercise includes the general purpose of the exercise, set-up, suggested repetitions and a reminder of how to properly execute the exercise. The general purpose reminds you why you are doing an exercise, so that you will perform it better. Through your study, you will be able to expand on the general purpose of the exercise for your own body. The set-up will remind you how to approach the exercise safely and efficiently. The number of repetitions is included as a general guideline because it is easy to forget that less is more in Pilates. It is better to do fewer repetitions with intensity, rather than many repetitions with poor form. A reminder of how to properly execute the exercise is included as a starting point for your own personal notes.

The most important part of this book will be written by you in the place for personal notes included with every exercise. With the help of your certified Pilates instructor, you will be able to write down your current modifications, helpful cue words, and useful imagery. Be sure to write your notes in pencil, as your notes will change as your body changes. There is no end to learning Pilates. Learn to savor each moment and each progression in your Pilates education. Then you will find yourself getting to the heart of the Method.

Pilates Review

The Pilates Method is more than a set of exercises. Joseph Pilates emphasized the importance of integrating mindfulness into the exercises to increase muscle control. He developed a method that connects the exercises of the matwork with the apparatus work to create a complete system of physical and mental conditioning for power and flexibility. It is a method that Joseph Pilates carefully constructed based on what has come to be known as Pilates principles. In order to get the most from your lessons with your Pilates instructor and from your home-based Pilates routine, it is essential that you understand the principles that form the foundation for the Pilates Method and the terminology used by your Pilates instructor. Your Pilates lessons have already exposed you to these Pilates concepts, they are included here as a reminder.

Pilates Principles

BREATHING
Breathing correctly with complete inhalations and exhalations revitalizes your body. Ideally, all breathing in Pilates is done through your nose, not your mouth, to avoid collapsing in your powerhouse. It is your breath that gives your exercises rhythm and helps you work more deeply.

CENTERING
Pilates focuses on proper alignment working within the frame of your body. Keeping movement within the frame of your body requires a lot of body control. You may be tempted to close your eyes to help you focus on an exercise, but Pilates requires outer awareness as well as inner awareness. Observe your body placement as you do your exercises to make sure that what feels centered truly is centered.

CONCENTRATION
Pilates is mind-body exercise. It incorporates what Pilates calls the five parts of the mind; intelligence, intuition, imagination, will and memory. Whereas music is often played in gyms as a form of distraction from mindless and repetitive movement, music is never played in a Pilates studio because total concentration is necessary in order to reap the full benefit of the movement. At an advanced level, Pilates can be a form of meditation.

CONTROL
Joseph Pilates called the Pilates system "Contrology" to describe the way in which the mind should control the muscles. All movements and positions are performed deliberately with mindfulness. Moving with control not only increases precision, but also avoids injury.

FLOW
Creating the maximum effect through a minimum of motion is the Pilates principle of flow. When Pilates is performed correctly, it gives you energy, it does not drain your energy. Moving your body intentionally, without adding any extra body adjustments, creates fluidity of movement. One of the hardest Pilates principles to master, moving with fluidity will take your Pilates practice to the highest level. It is where the science of Pilates becomes an art form.

PRECISION
It is the attention to details that makes Pilates a lifetime practice. Pilates never ends, there will always be more to refine and a higher level to aspire to. This is what makes Pilates so intriguing. The key is to learn to savor each moment, and focus on each progression.

Pilates Terms

ANCHORING THE SPINE
Anchoring the spine refers to the placement of your back when it touches a surface such as the mat, the reformer carriage or the wall. Use the image of "buttoning" your belly button to the mat to help you engage your stomach muscles. Gently pressing your spine into the mat (without exaggerating the movement to the point of tucking your pelvis), will allow you to move your limbs freely, without the danger of transferring the work into your back instead of your powerhouse.

C-CURVE
The c-curve is a movement initiated from your abdominals that creates a "C" shape in your back. It strengthens your stomach while it stretches your lower back. To avoid collapsing into your waistline, imagine creating an uppercase letter "C" with your whole torso, instead of a lower case letter "c" with your lower back.

FRAME
The frame is the box made by "connecting the four dots" from shoulder to shoulder and hip to hip.

LENGTHENING THE NECK
Lengthening your neck helps keep tension out of your neck and shoulders so that you can concentrate on your powerhouse. It is a cue that refers to elongating the back of your neck, not the front of your throat. When lying down, keep your chin low (without forcing your chin to your chest) and press the back of your neck gently into the mat. It may be necessary to place a thin pillow under your head to achieve the proper neck placement. When sitting or standing, keep your gaze straight ahead with your chin tilted down slightly and lift upwards from the base of your skull. Imagine you are being lifted from your ears.

LIFTING THE POWERHOUSE
Lifting the powerhouse is a technique used to engage your stomach muscles by pulling your belly button in and up, as if zipping up tight pants. This one concept alone can improve your posture.

PILATES STANCE
Pilates stance is a slight rotation of your legs at your hips. As the top of your thighs rotate outwards from one another, the back of your thighs come towards each other, bringing your heels together. This position helps keep the work in your powerhouse and it shapes your legs. It is not a position that is available to everyone (for example, some people, such as those with knock knees, may be better off working with the legs parallel apart).

POWERHOUSE
The powerhouse is your control center. It includes your stomach, top of your inner thighs and bottom. To work your body safely and get positive results from your workouts, it is imperative that you engage your powerhouse.

SCOOPING THE STOMACH
Scooping the stomach describes the way you hollow out your abdominals as you pull your belly button in towards your spine.

SUPPORTING SIDE
Supporting side refers to the side of the body that remains isolated while other body parts are in motion. Although stationary, the muscles in the supporting leg, hip and side of the torso are engaged, thus allowing the working leg to execute the movement.

WORKING HEIGHT
Working height refers to the proper placement of your legs in the air when performing exercises lying on your back. Your legs are at the correct level when your abdominals are engaged, and there is no strain in your neck or back.

WORKING LEG
The working leg is the leg that is in motion during the exercise.

WRAPPING THE THIGHS
Wrapping the thighs is a further description of the Pilates stance. Imagine each leg as a candy cane with the stripes spiraling away from each other to draw the back of your thighs and heels together with your insteps lifted.

WRINGING OUT THE LUNGS
Wringing out the lungs uses the analogy of wringing out a wet towel to help you squeeze the last drop of air out of your lungs as you twist from your waistline.

The Basic Matwork

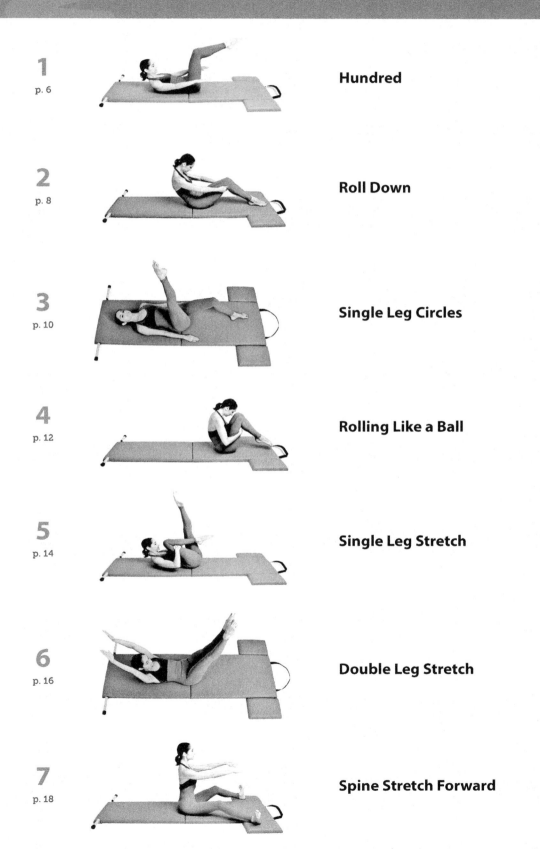

1
p. 6

Hundred

2
p. 8

Roll Down

3
p. 10

Single Leg Circles

4
p. 12

Rolling Like a Ball

5
p. 14

Single Leg Stretch

6
p. 16

Double Leg Stretch

7
p. 18

Spine Stretch Forward

Hundred

General Purpose:
The hundred warms up the body and improves endurance.

Set-up:
Lie down on your back and draw your knees into your chest.

Repetitions:
10 sets.

Reminder:
With so much to focus on while performing the hundred (head position, arm movement, breathing, counting, leg position…), it is advisable to practice only one or two components of the hundred in the early phases of learning it, then slowly build up to the full exercise.

My Notes:

a.

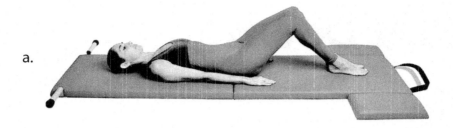

b.

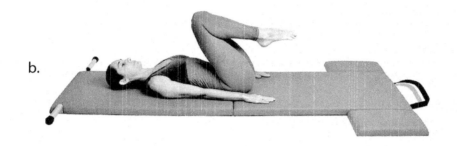

c.

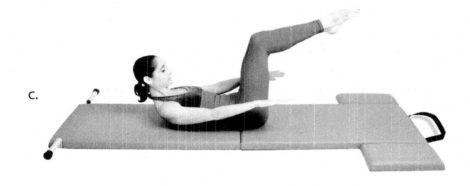

d.

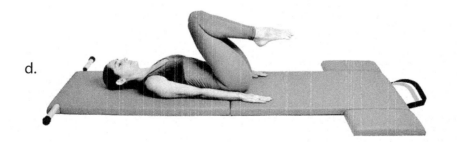

Roll Down

General Purpose:
The roll down strengthens the powerhouse and develops articulation of the spine.

Set-up:
Turn to your side to sit up and face the front of the mat. Keep your feet on the mat with bent legs together. Place your hands lightly behind your thighs.

Repetitions:
3-5 times.

Reminder:
Keep a light touch on your legs to avoid doing the work with your arms instead of your powerhouse. Start out with a small range of movement and gradually increase the range as your strength improves.

My Notes:

For added safety, secure your feet under a foot strap or a low piece of furniture.

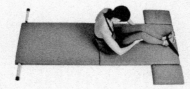

a.

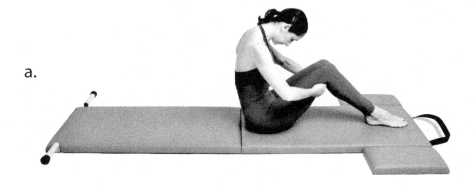

b.

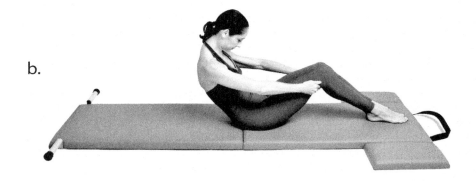

c.

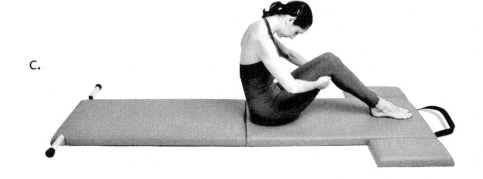

Single Leg Circles

General Purpose:
The single leg circles develop stability in the torso while moving the leg at the hip.

Set-up:
Lie down with your legs bent and your feet placed hip width apart on the mat. Draw one knee to your chest and extend that same leg up for the circles.

Repetitions:
5 circles and reverse with each leg.

Reminder:
The first set of leg circles always start across the body.

My Notes:

Detail

Bending your bottom leg will help you increase the stretch in your raised leg and provide you with more stability in your torso.

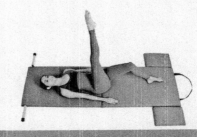

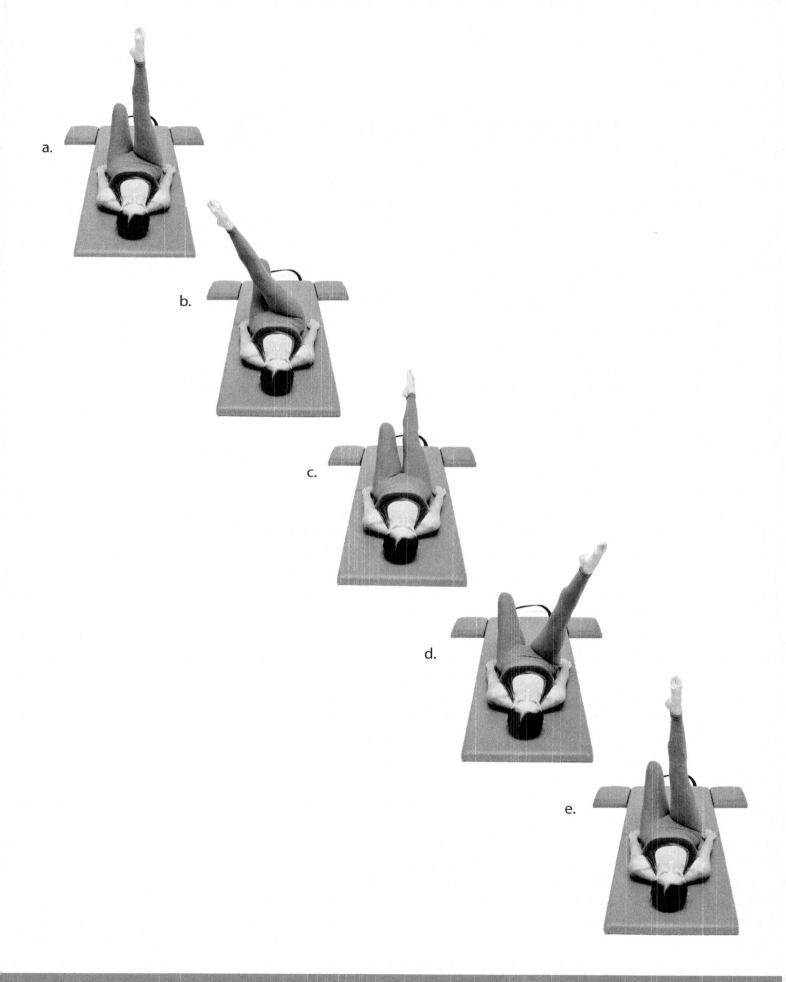

Rolling Like a Ball

General Purpose:
Rolling like a ball improves balance control and powerhouse strength, and massages the pressure points along both sides of the spine.

Set-up:
Turn to your side to sit up and face the front of the mat. Place your hands on the mat next to your hips and with your weight distributed between your hands and feet lift your seat forward towards the front end of the mat. Take a seat by your feet and place your hands behind your thighs with your chin towards your chest.

Repetitions:
6 times.

Reminder:
Try to master the balance with your toes off the mat before adding the rolling movement.

My Notes:

Transition into rolling like a ball

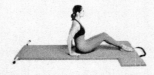
a.

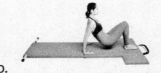
b.

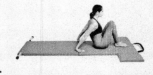
c.

a.

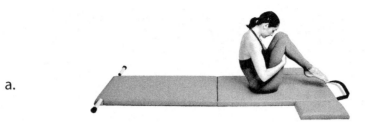

b.

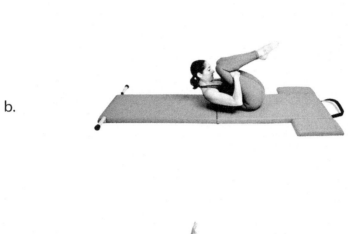

c.

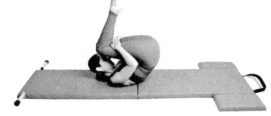

d.

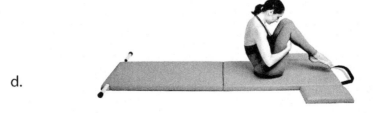

Single Leg Stretch

General Purpose:
The single leg stretch strengthens the powerhouse and stretches the back.

Set-up:
Place your hands behind you on the mat and lift your seat back towards the center of the mat. Hug one leg with both hands stacked behind your thigh. Lie down with the leg you are holding bent to your chest while the other leg lengthens out in front of you in Pilates stance. If it is available to you, leave your head up, otherwise, rest it on pillows.

Repetitions:
6-10 times.

Reminder:
Keep your elbows lifted to work your underarms.

My Notes:

Detail

Transition into the single leg stretch

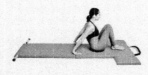
a.

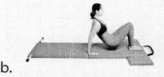
b.

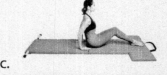
c.

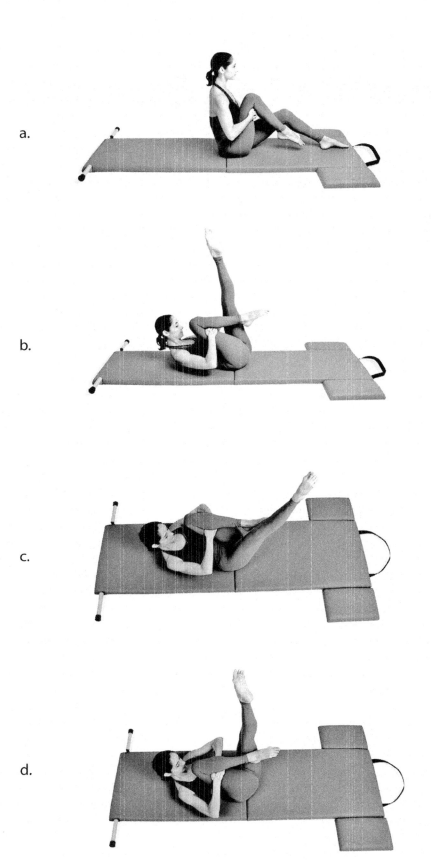

a.

b.

c.

d.

Double Leg Stretch

General Purpose:
The double leg stretch strengthens the powerhouse and improves coordination and breathing.

Set-up:
Draw both knees into your chest and place your hands behind your thighs. If it is available to you, leave your head up, otherwise, rest it on pillows.

Repetitions:
5 times.

Reminder:
In the beginning stages of learning the double leg stretch, leave out the arm movement. When you are ready to add the arms, remember that your legs stay together as your arms circle open.

My Notes:

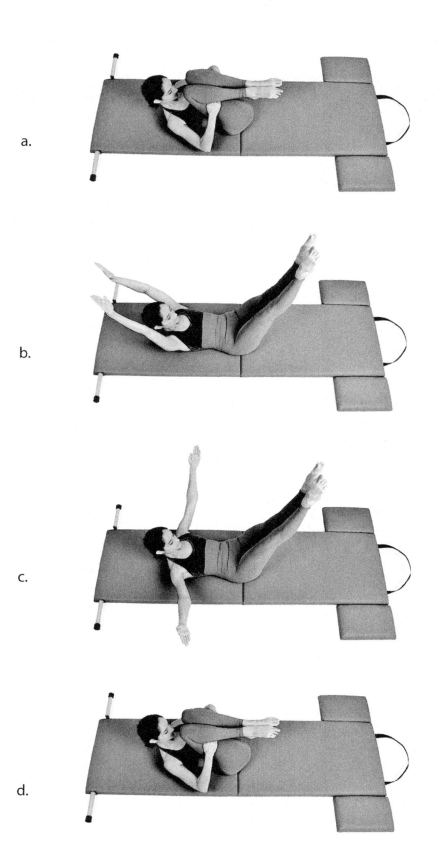

a.

b.

c.

d.

Spine Stretch Forward

General Purpose:
The spine stretch forward stretches the spine and the back of the legs, and emphasizes the emptying of the lungs.

Set-up:
Turn to your side to sit up and face the front of the mat. Extend your legs a little wider than your mat, flex your feet and sit tall. Extend your arms out in front of you at shoulder height and shoulder width apart.

Repetitions:
3 times.

Reminder:
If it is hard for you to sit tall, let your knees bend a little.

My Notes:

a.

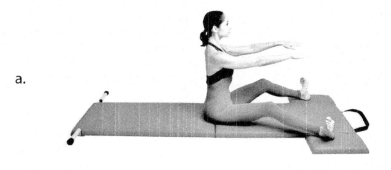

b.

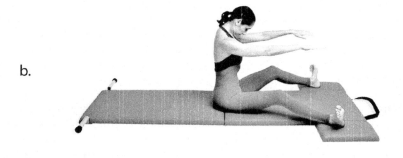

c.

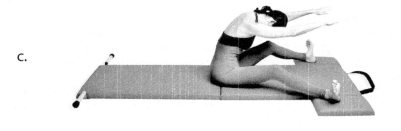

d.

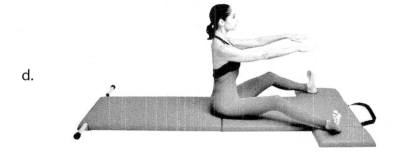

The Intermediate Matwork

1
p. 24

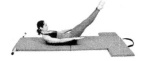

Hundred

2
p. 26

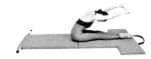

Roll-Up

3
p. 28

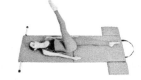

Single Leg Circles

4
p. 30

Rolling Like a Ball

5
p. 32

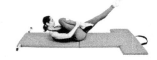

Single Leg Stretch

6
p. 34

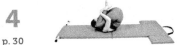

Double Leg Stretch

7
p. 36

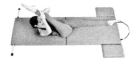

Single Straight Leg

8
p. 38

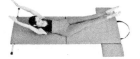

Double Straight Leg

9
p. 40

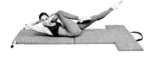

Criss Cross

10
p. 42

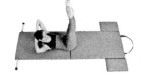

Spine Stretch Forward

11
(p. 44)
p. 46

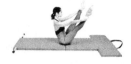

Open Leg Rocker

12
p. 48

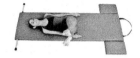

Corkscrew

13
p. 50

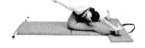

Saw

14
p. 52

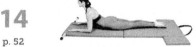

Neck Roll

15
p. 54

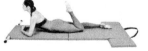

Single Leg Kicks

16
p. 56

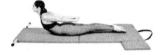

Double Leg Kicks

17
p. 60

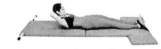

Neck Pull

18
p. 62-69

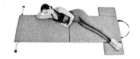

Side Leg Kick Series

19
(p. 70)
p. 72

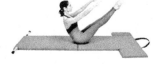

Teaser

20
p. 74

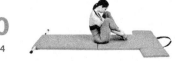

Seal

Standing Preparation

General Purpose:
To lower oneself to the floor with poise and control.

Set-up:
If it is available to you, stand at the front end of your mat and cross your feet and your arms to take a seat, otherwise, take a seat on the mat in the safest way possible for your body.

Repetitions:
1 time.

Reminder:
Pull your belly button in and up as you lower yourself to the ground.

My Notes:

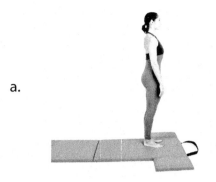

a.

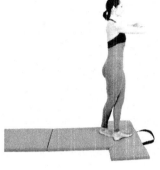

b.

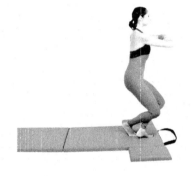

c.

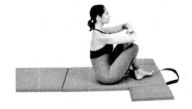

d.

Transition from the standing preparation into the matwork:

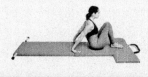

a.

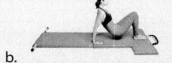

b.

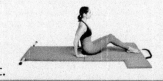

c.

Hundred

General Purpose:
The hundred warms up the body and improves endurance.

Set-up:
Lie down on your back and draw your knees into your chest.

Repetitions:
10 Sets.

Reminder:
The proper head and leg position will keep the work in your powerhouse and eliminate strain in your neck and back.

My Notes:

a.

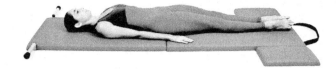

b.

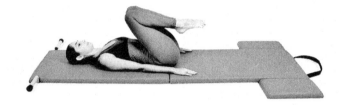

c.

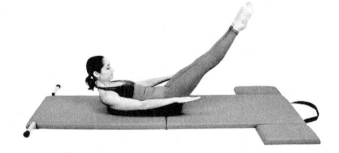

d.

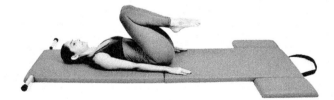

Roll-Up

General Purpose:
The roll-up strengthens the powerhouse and develops articulation of the spine.

Set-up:
Lengthen your legs out on the mat in Pilates stance as your arms stretch up and slightly back. The use of a bar between your hands is a great option for keeping your arms even. A weighted bar is a great option for opening your chest and shoulders before rolling up, and a great way to counterbalance the weight of your legs as you roll up to sitting.

Repetitions:
3-5 times.

Reminder:
Start with your arms at the proper height above the mat to help anchor your spine. You may need to hold the back of your legs and/or use a foot strap to avoid using momentum as you sit up.

My Notes:

Keep your heels together as you perform the roll-up.

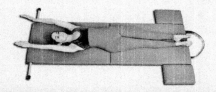

a.

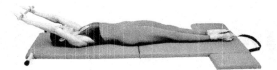

b.

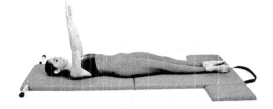

c.

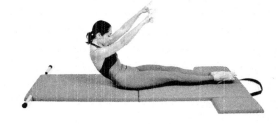

d.

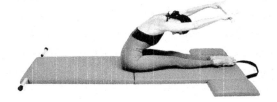

e.

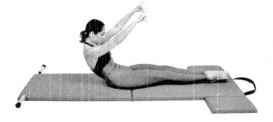

Single Leg Circles

General Purpose:
The single leg circles develop stability in the torso while moving the leg at the hip.

Set-up:
After lying down, lift one leg up in the air in Pilates stance.

Repetitions:
5 circles and reverse with each leg.

Reminder:
If tension gets into your neck, bend your supporting leg with your foot on the mat, and/or use a pillow under your head.

My Notes:

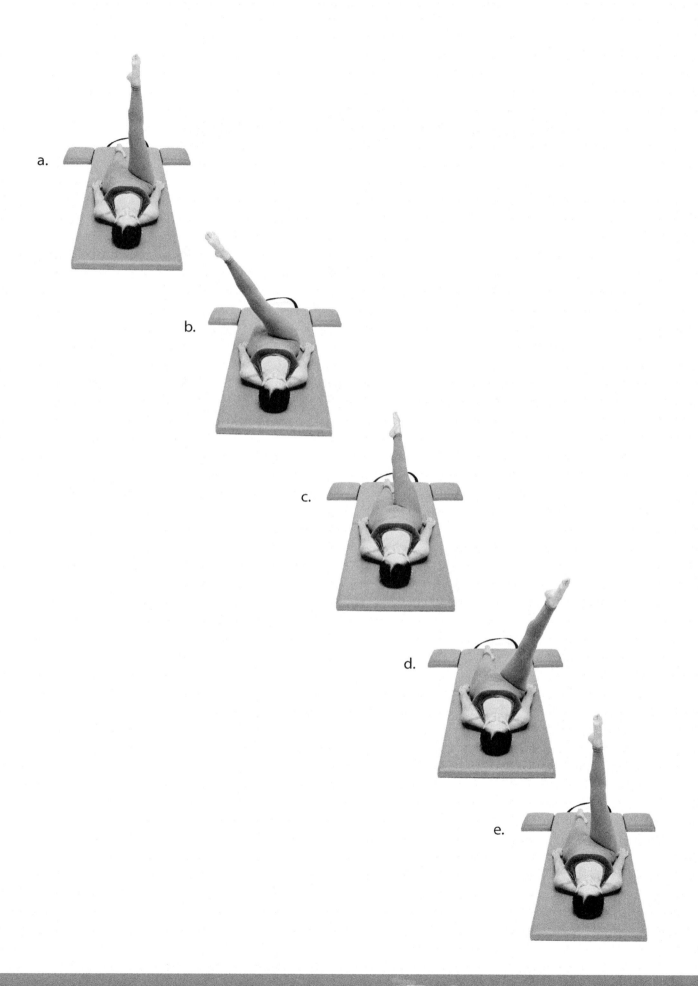

a.

b.

c.

d.

e.

Rolling Like a Ball

General Purpose:
Rolling like a ball improves balance control and powerhouse strength, and massages the pressure points along both sides of the spine.

Set-up:
Sit up carefully and place your hands on the mat by your hips. With your weight distributed between your hands and feet, lift your seat forward towards the front end of the mat. Take a seat by your feet and place your hands on the outside of your ankles with your chin towards your chest.

Repetitions:
6 times.

Reminder:
Try to keep your nose between your knees, your thighs close to your chest and your feet near your seat throughout the exercise. Rolling like a ball is one of the most challenging exercises in the matwork series.

My Notes:

Detail

Transition into rolling like a ball

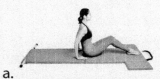

a.

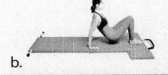

b.

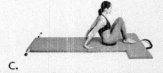

c.

a.

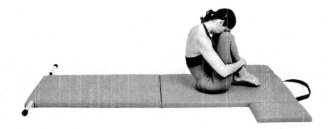

b.

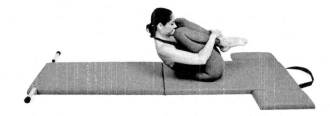

c.

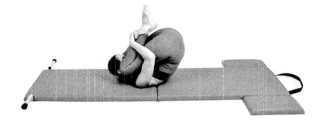

d.

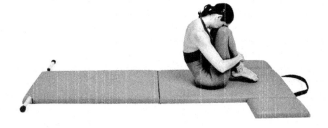

Place your hands on each ankle to keep your feet close to your seat.

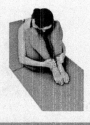

For more of a challenge, place your hands in a "basket weave" with your left hand on your right ankle and your right hand on your left wrist.

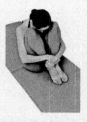

Single Leg Stretch

General Purpose:
The single leg stretch strengthens the powerhouse and stretches the back.

Set-up:
Place your hands behind you on the mat and lift your seat back towards the center of the mat. Hug one leg to your chest with the hand matching the bent leg on your ankle and the opposite hand just below your knee on your shin. Lie down with the bent leg to your chest while the other leg lengthens out in front of you in Pilates stance. If it is available to you, leave your head up, otherwise rest it on pillows.

Repetitions:
6-10 times.

Reminder:
The correct hand placement on your bent leg not only develops your coordination, it also improves the alignment of your shoulder, knee, hip and ankle.

My Notes:

Transition into the single leg stretch

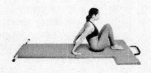

a.

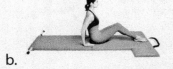

b.

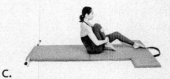

c.

a.

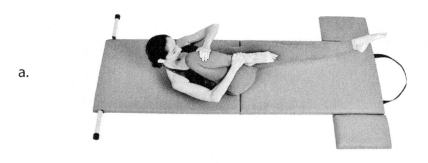

b.

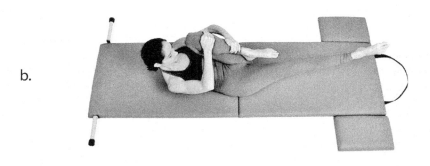

c.

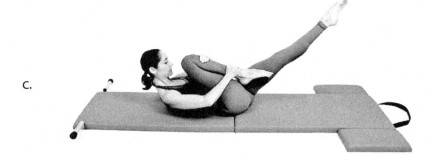

d.

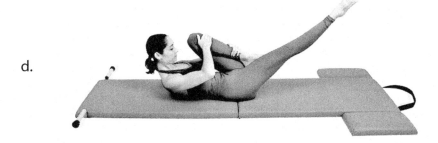

Double Leg Stretch

General Purpose:
The double leg stretch strengthens the powerhouse and improves coordination and breathing.

Set-up:
Draw both knees into your chest and place your hands on your ankles. If it is available to you, leave your head up, otherwise rest it on pillows.

Repetitions:
5 times.

Reminder:
If keeping your head lifted is available to you, be sure to isolate your head position from the movement in your arms and legs.

My Notes:

a.

b.

c.

d.

Single Straight Leg

General Purpose:
The single straight leg strengthens the powerhouse, stretches the back of the raised leg and stretches the front of the hip of the bottom leg.

Set-up:
Extend one leg up towards the sky and hold it with both hands. Extend your other leg out in front of you just a few inches above the mat. If it is available to you, leave your head up, otherwise rest it on pillows.

Repetitions:
6-10 times.

Reminder:
Stack your hands evenly above or below the back of the knee of your raised leg (be sure not to grab directly behind your knee). Be sure your **bottom leg does not rest on the mat.**

My Notes:

Keep your bottom leg a few inches above the mat to maximize the stretch in the front of your hip.

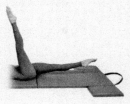

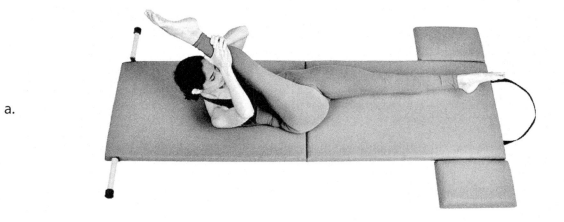

a.

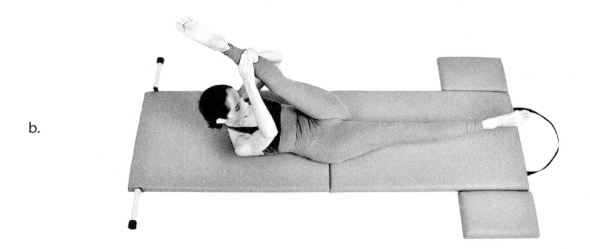

b.

Double Straight Leg

General Purpose:
The double straight leg deepens the powerhouse strength.

Set-up:
Extend both legs up to the sky in Pilates stance and stack your hands behind your head. If it is available to you, leave your head up, otherwise rest it on pillows.

Repetitions:
5 times.

Reminder:
Inhale as your legs lower and exhale as they lift. The accent is on the up beat.

My Notes:

a.

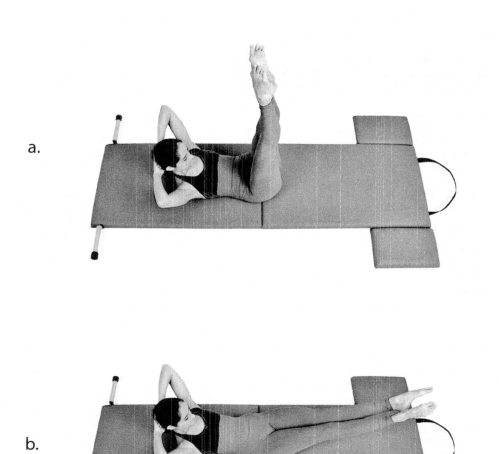

b.

c.

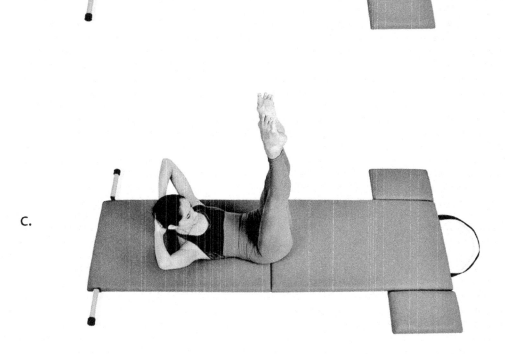

Criss Cross

General Purpose:
The criss cross works the waistline and wrings the air out of the lungs.

Set-up:
Bend one knee to your chest and extend your other leg to working height. Keep your hands stacked behind your head with your elbows open wide.

Repetitions:
1-3 sets

Reminder:
Exhale during each twist for 3 counts before twisting to your other side.

My Notes:

a.

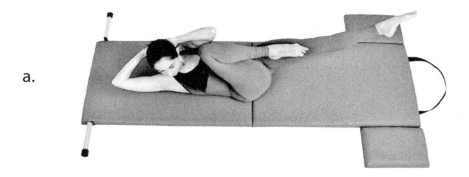

b.

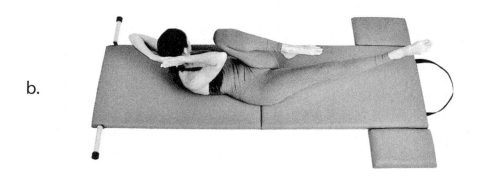

c.

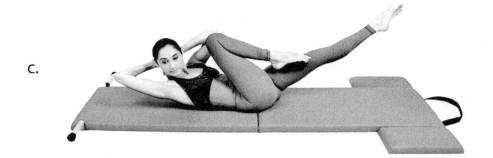

Spine Stretch Forward

General Purpose:
The spine stretch forward stretches the spine and the back of the legs, and emphasizes the emptying of the lungs.

Set-up:
Sit up carefully and extend your legs a little wider than your mat and flex your feet. Sit tall and extend your arms out in front of you at shoulder height and shoulder width apart.

Repetitions:
3 times.

Reminder:
Emphasize the exhale as you bend forward and bury the top of your head into your stomach.

My Notes:

a.

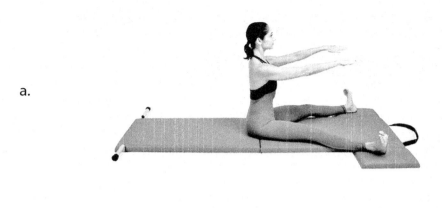

b.

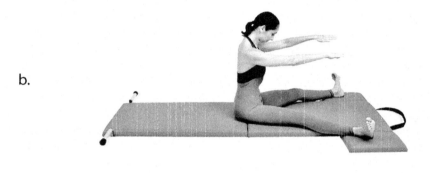

c.

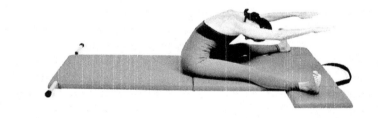

d.

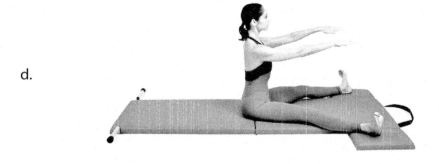

Open Leg Rocker Preparation

General Purpose:
The open leg rocker preparation improves balance control and powerhouse strength, and limbers the back of the legs.

Set-up:
Bend your legs and draw your toes together in front of you. Grab your ankles and extend your legs out towards the top corners of the room.

Repetitions:
3 sets.

Reminder:
Once you have mastered the balance control on this exercise, you can skip it and go directly into the rolling open leg rocker.

My Notes:

Detail

To increase the flexibility in the back of your legs, wrap a neck tie or strap around each foot.

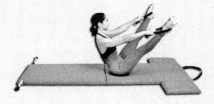

a.

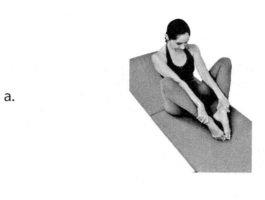

b.

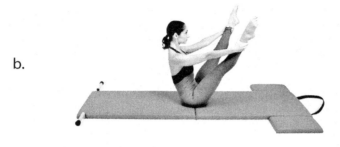

c.

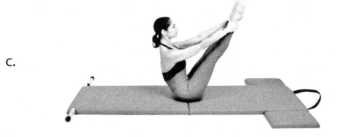

d.

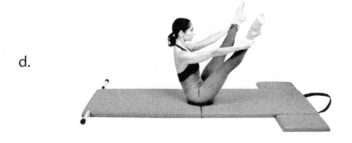

e.

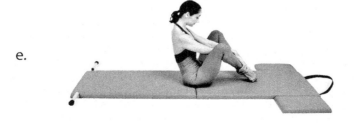

Open Leg Rocker

General Purpose:
The open leg rocker improves balance control and powerhouse strength, limbers the back of the legs, and massages the pressure points along both sides of the spine.

Set-up:
Bend your legs and draw your toes together in front of you. Grab your ankles and extend your legs out towards the top corners of the room.

Repetitions:
6 times.

Reminder:
Keep your arms long while rolling.

My Notes:

Detail

To deepen your c-curve prior to extending your legs, keep your arms long as you hold your ankles and pull your waist away from your toes.

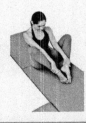

a.

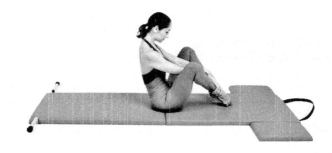

b.

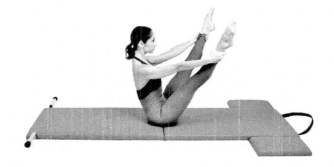

c.

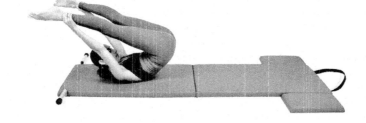

d.

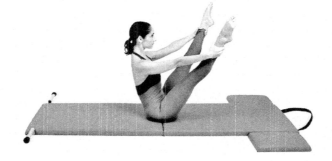

Corkscrew

General Purpose:
The corkscrew strengthens the sides of the body and deepens the powerhouse strength.

Set-up:
After the open leg rocker, draw your legs together straight and slide your hands down the back of your legs as you lie down. Rest your arms by your side and keep your legs extended up towards the sky.

Repetitions:
6 times.

Reminder:
Keep your heels even and together with your ankle bones slightly apart throughout the exercise.

My Notes:

Transition into the corkscrew

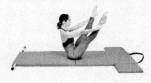
a.

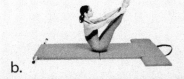
b.

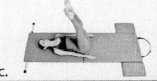
c.

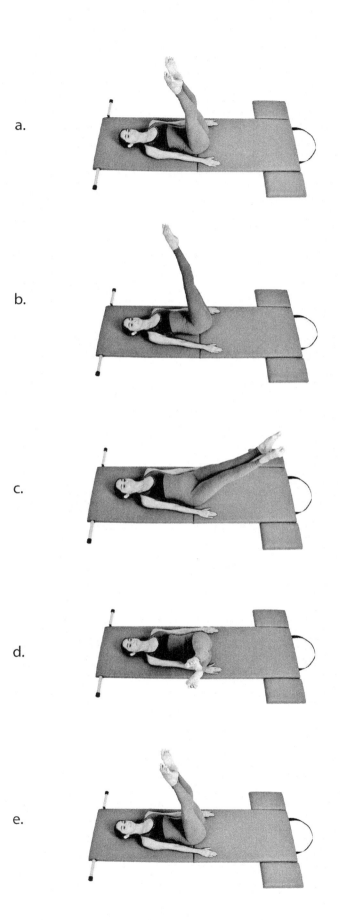

Saw

General Purpose:
The saw works the waistline, wrings the air out of the lungs, opens the lower back, and stretches the back of the legs.

Set-up:
Sit up carefully and extend your legs a little wider than your mat. Flex your feet and sit tall with your arms extended out to the side.

Repetitions:
4 times.

Reminder:
Keep your hips anchored to the mat as your little finger reaches to the outside of your little toe on your opposite foot.

My Notes:

a.

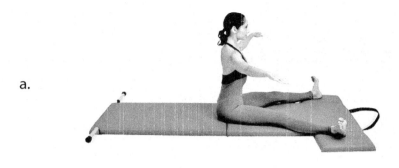

b.

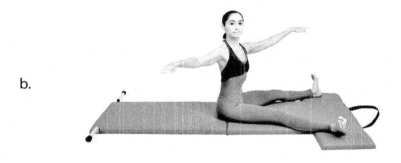

c.

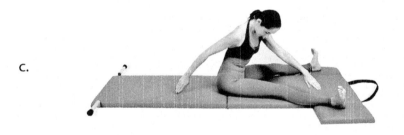

d.

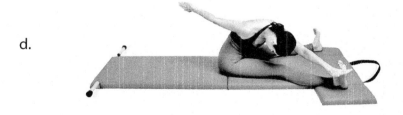

Neck Roll

General Purpose:
The neck roll stretches the neck and opens the chest.

Set-up:
Bring your legs together and turn to your stomach. Prop yourself up on your elbows (or push up to straight arms if it is available to you).

Repetitions:
2 times.

Reminder:
Keep your belly button off the mat throughout the exercise.

My Notes:

Detail

To facilitate pushing up to straight arms on the neck roll, hold the dowels on the outside of the mat. For a deeper stretch, position your shoulders closer to the edge of the mat and push up to straight arms, perpendicular to the mat.

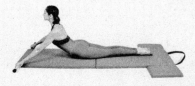

a.

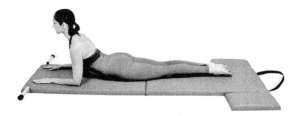

b.

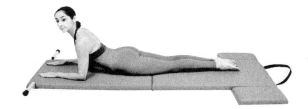

c.

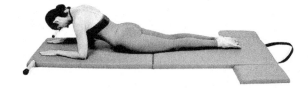

d.

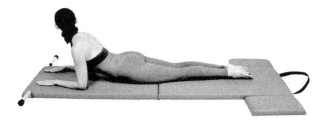

e.

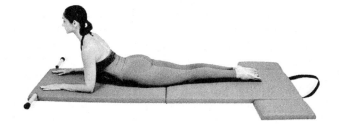

Single Leg Kicks

General Purpose:
The single leg kicks stretch the front of the hips and top of the thighs while strengthening the seat and back of the legs.

Set-up:
Place your elbows directly under your shoulders and make fists with your knuckles touching each other.

Repetitions:
10 times.

Reminder:
Keep your feet loose and your seat tight during the double pulse of each leg.

My Notes:

a.

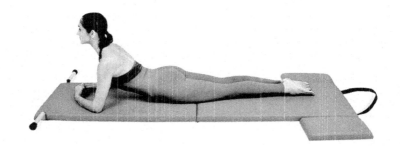

b.

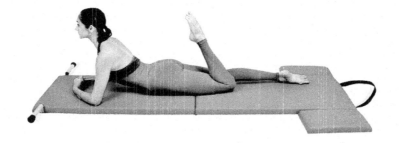

c.

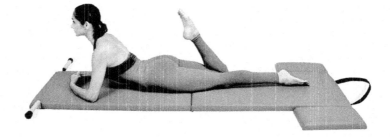

Double Leg Kicks

General Purpose:
The double leg kicks strengthen the back of the legs and open the chest and shoulders.

Set-up:
Stack your hands high on your back with bent arms and your palms facing the sky. Turn your head to one side and rest it on the mat.

Repetitions:
4 times.

Reminder:
Pulse your feet together three times before lifting your chest. Your arms and legs should stretch simultaneously.

My Notes:

a.

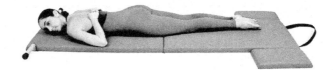

b.

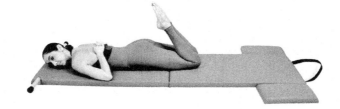

c.

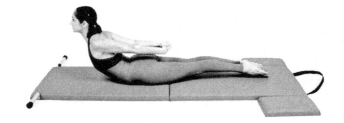

d.

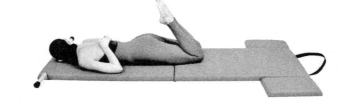

Counter Stretch

General Purpose:
The counter stretch opens the lower back.

Set-up:
Sit back towards your heels, lower you head and scoop your stomach.

Repetitions:
1 time.

Reminder:
If this position is not available to you, turn to your back and gently pull your knees into your chest.

My Notes:

a.

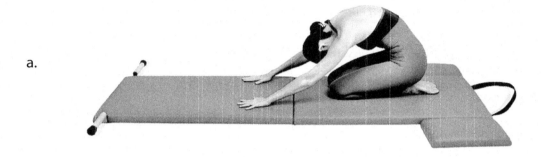

b.

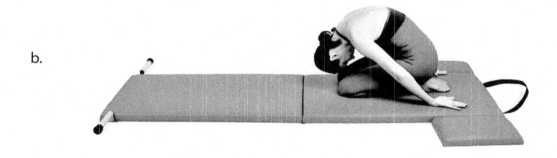

Neck Pull

General Purpose:
The neck pull deepens the powerhouse strength and develops articulation of the spine.

Set-up:
Carefully turn to your back. Lie down with your hands stacked behind your head and elbows wide. Legs are hip width apart, parallel, with flexed feet.

Repetitions:
3-5 times.

Reminder:
Stay round to come up. Roll up to a straight back before lying down. For more of a challenge, you can add a hinge with a flat back before rolling down on the mat.

My Notes:

If at any point during your neck pull you antici-pate using momentum instead of powerhouse strength, try placing your hands behind your thighs to help you articulate your spine and keep the work in your powerhouse. This modification is especially helpful if you are still using a foot strap in the studio, but do not have one available for your home practice.

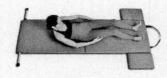

a.

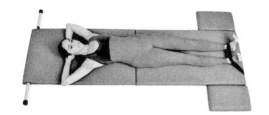

b.

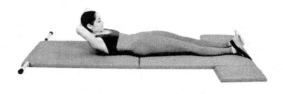

c.

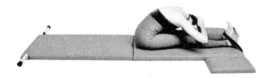

d.

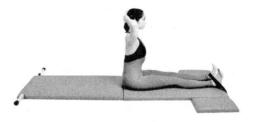

e.

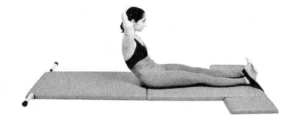

f.

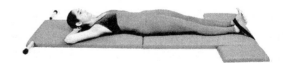

Side Leg Kick Series: Front / Back

General Purpose:
The front/back side leg kick series develops torso control while moving the working leg. The kick to the front stretches the back of the leg and the kick to the back opens the front of the hip.

Set-up:
Turn to one side and line your elbow, shoulder, waist and hip with the back edge of the mat. Prop your head up with your hand, place your other hand on the mat in front of your waist, and keep your gaze straight ahead. Lengthen your legs and rest your feet off the front edge of the mat.

Repetitions:
8-10 times.

Reminder:
Before starting the kicks, turn your top leg out at your hip, lengthen it beyond your bottom leg, and lift it to working hip height.

My Notes:

Detail

Alternate set-up: Lengthen your bottom arm long in front of you and rest your head on pillows.

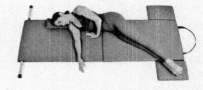

a.

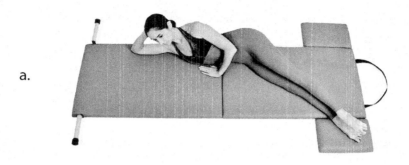

b.

c.

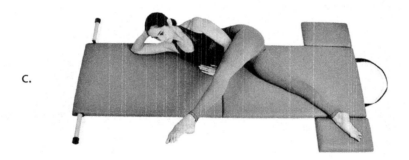

d.

Side Leg Kick Series: Up / Down

General Purpose:
The up/down side leg kick series develops torso control while toning the working leg. The outer thigh is strengthened as the working leg lifts, and the inner thigh is strengthened as the working leg comes down.

Set-up:
Same set up as side leg kick series: front/back.

Repetitions:
5 times.

Reminder:
Keep your top leg hovering directly over your bottom leg. Focus on good form rather than the height of your leg.

My Notes:

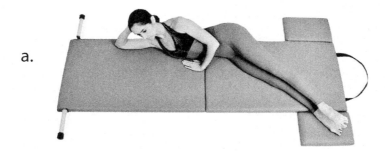

a.

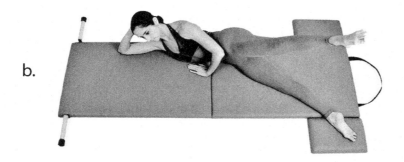

b.

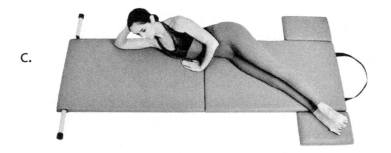

c.

Side Leg Kick Series: Circles

General Purpose:
The circles in the side leg kick series develop torso control and shape the thigh of the circling leg.

Set-up:
Same set up as side leg kick series: front/back.

Repetitions:
5 circles and reverse.

Reminder:
Strike your heels on each circle and keep your ankle bones lifted.

My Notes:

a.

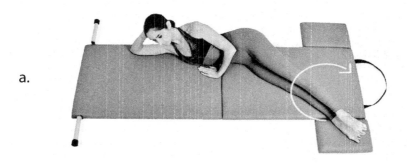

b.

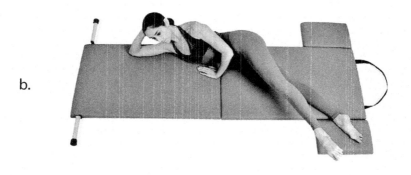

c.

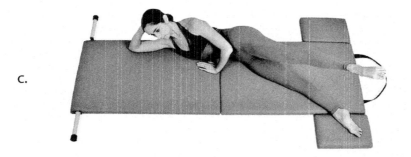

d.

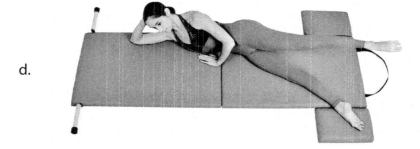

Heel Beats

General Purpose:
The heel beats strengthen the seat and back of legs, and provide an efficient transition into the side leg kick series on the other side.

Set-up:
Turn to your stomach and rest your forehead on your hands.

Repetitions:
3 sets of ten heel beats.

Reminder:
Pull your stomach in to keep pressure out of your lower back. After the heel beats, turn to your other side, and repeat the side leg kick series on your second side.

My Notes:

a.

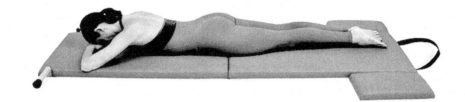

b.

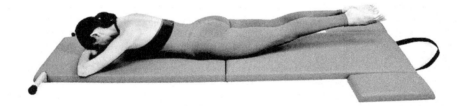

Teaser Preparation

General Purpose:
The teaser preparation develops powerhouse strength while providing support for the feet.

Set-up:
Sit facing a wall and place your feet together, parallel on the wall. Your toes should be about eye level, and your legs should be bent at an angle slightly more than 90 degrees.

Repetitions:
3 times.

Reminder:
Use your feet to push into the wall as you roll your back into the floor and as you roll up again. You can start out with a small movement in your torso and work up to the full range of movement that goes all the way to the floor. You may need to have someone spot your feet during the exercise. When your powerhouse is strong enough, skip this preparation and go directly into the teaser exercise.

My Notes:

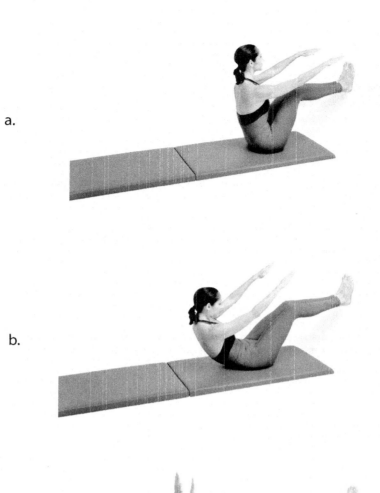

a.

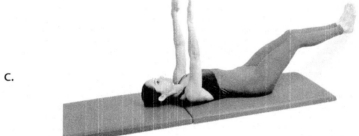

b.

c.

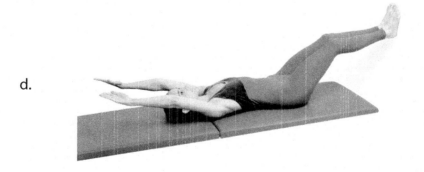

d.

Teaser

General Purpose:
The teaser deepens the powerhouse strength, develops articulation of the spine, and works the balance control.

Set-up:
Lie down on your back and draw your knees into your chest. As your legs extend forward into the air in a Pilates stance, extend your arms straight back above the mat in the opposite direction. Be sure your back is anchored to the mat through your stomach.

Repetitions:
3 times.

Reminder:
To avoid momentum, you can place your hands on the back of your legs as you sit up. To improve the c-curve in your torso, it may be necessary to bend your legs into a table top position with your legs together parallel.

My Notes:

a.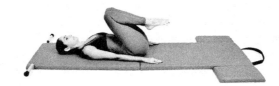

b.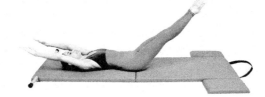

c.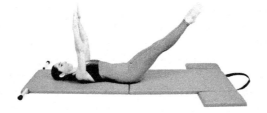

d.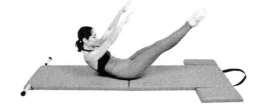

e.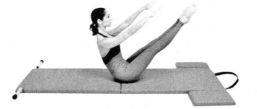

Seal

General Purpose:
The seal is a cool down exercise that improves balance control and powerhouse strength, massages the pressure points along both sides of the spine, and develops coordination.

Set-up:
Sit up carefully and interlace your arms through the <u>inside</u> of your legs and wrap your hands on the <u>outside</u> of your ankles.

Repetitions:
6 times.

Reminder:
Click your insteps together instead of clicking the soles of your feet together. Clicking the insteps will keep your knees more within your frame, which will deepen your c-curve and deepen the work in your stomach and inner thighs.

My Notes:

Detail

Starting position for the seal

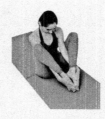

a.

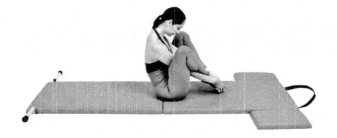

b.

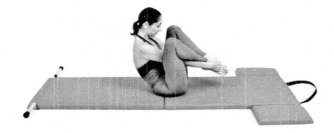

c.

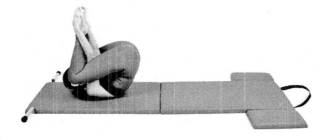

d.

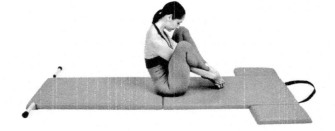

Standing Finish

General Purpose:
Standing up from the seated seal position strengthens the seat and legs and improves balance control.

Set-up:
If it is available to you, cross your feet and stand up after the last repetition of the seal exercise.

Repetitions:
1 time.

Reminder:
Skip the clicks of your insteps when you roll back on the last set of the seal (the sixth set), and use that extra time to unlace your arms from your legs and cross your feet, thus improving your timing as you stand up.

My Notes:

a.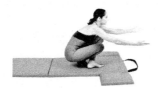

b.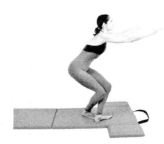

c.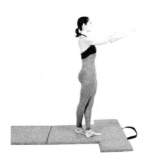

d.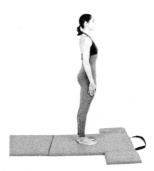

The Magic Circle Matwork

1
p. 82
p. 84

Hundred

2
p. 86

Roll-Up

3
p. 88

Single Leg Circles

4
p. 90

Rolling Like a Ball

5
p. 92

Double Leg Stretch

6
p. 94

Double Straight Leg

7
p. 96

Criss Cross

8
p. 98

Single Leg Stretch

9
p. 100

Single Straight Leg

10
p. 102
p. 104

Spine Stretch Forward

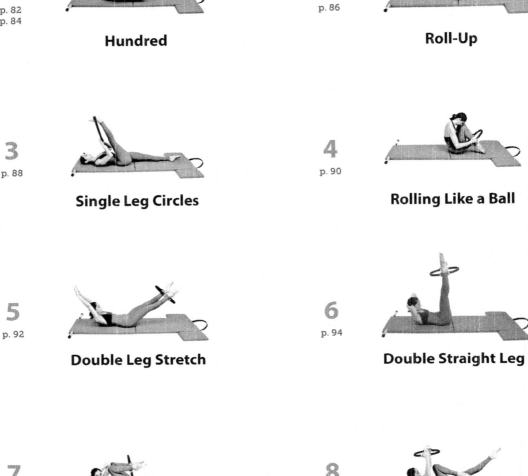
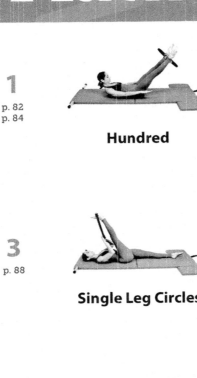
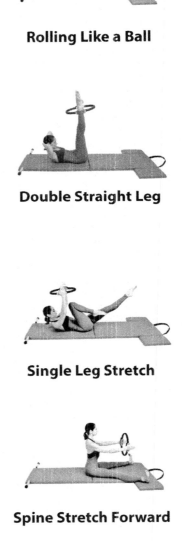
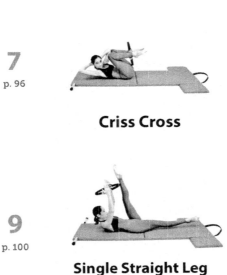

11
p. 106

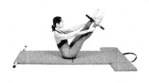

Open Leg Rocker

12
p. 108

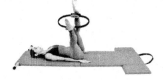

Corkscrew

13
p. 110

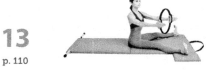

Saw

14
p. 112

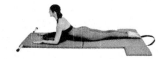

Neck Roll

15
p. 114

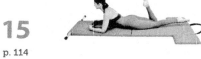

Single Leg Kicks

16
p. 116

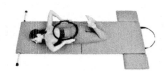

Double Leg Kicks

17
p. 118
p. 120

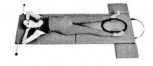

Neck Pull

18
p. 122-129

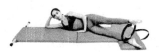

Side Leg Series

19
p. 130
p. 132

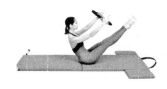

Teaser

20
p. 134

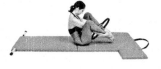

Seal

About Using The Magic Circle In The Matwork

This section outlines just a few of the many ways to incorporate the magic circle into your matwork practice. Once you have developed a good understanding of the regular matwork, the magic circle will add variety to your Pilates workouts and help you deepen the work in your stomach, bottom and inner thighs. The goal is to be able to transfer the same intensity used with the circle into your regular matwork routine.

In general, the order of the matwork stays the same when using the circle, but when doing the series of five with the circle, you can change the order to improve the flow. Grouping the double leg stretch, double straight leg and criss cross together (when the circle is between your ankles) and grouping the single leg stretch and single straight leg together (when the circle is between your hands) keeps the transitions more fluid.

Squeeze the circle without locking your elbows or knees to keep the work in your powerhouse. On the exercises where the magic circle can be used in more than one way (for example the hundred can be performed with the circle between your ankles or between your hands), pick the one variation that will benefit you the most. Using the circle intensifies every exercise, so incorporate the magic circle into only a few of the mat exercises to avoid overexertion. **It is not necessary to use the magic circle on every single exercise within the same workout.**

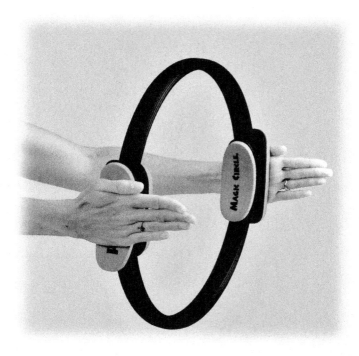

Magic Circle Hundred: Variation One

General Purpose:
The hundred warms up the body and improves endurance.

Set-up:
Lie down on your back and draw your knees into your chest with the circle in the palms of your hands.

Repetitions:
10 sets.

Reminder:
Pulse the circle for each count, keeping your arms just above your legs. As you get stronger, you can pulse the circle while raising your arms up to the sky (inhale), and pulse the circle as you lower your arms down towards your legs (exhale).

My Notes:

a.

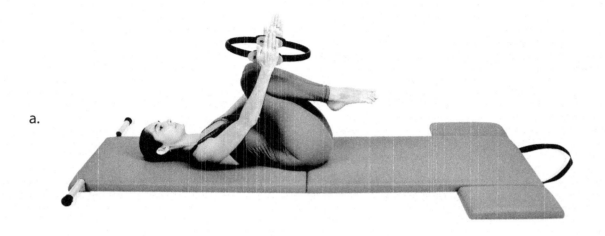

b.

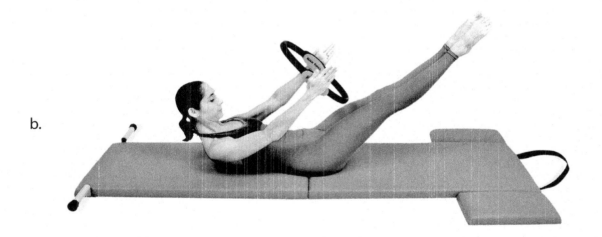

Magic Circle Hundred: Variation Two

General Purpose:
The hundred warms up the body and improves endurance.

Set-up:
Lie down on your back and draw your knees into your chest. Place the circle between your ankles.

Repetitions:
10 sets.

Reminder:
Squeeze with constant pressure on the circle. If your legs start to wobble, squeeze your seat more. The circle may not seem heavy at first but that may change as you progress through the exercise. To counterbalance the weight of the circle you may need to lift your legs higher.

My Notes:

a.

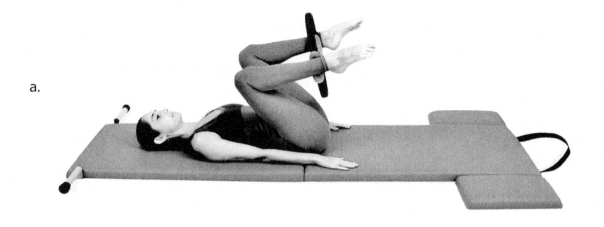

b.

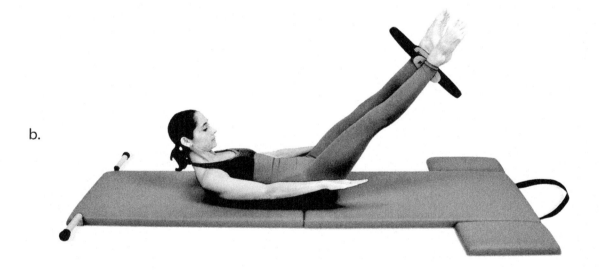

Magic Circle Roll-Up

General Purpose:
The roll-up strengthens the powerhouse and develops articulation of the spine.

Set-up:
Lengthen your legs out on the mat in Pilates stance as your arms stretch up and slightly back with the circle between the palms of your hands. If your back can stay anchored to the mat, place the edge of your circle on the mat behind you.

Repetitions:
3-5 times.

Reminder:
As you roll up, squeeze the circle on your inhale and release the pressure on your exhale, repeat the same pattern on the way down. Squeezing into the circle with long arms is a great way to keep the effort in your powerhouse and avoid momentum.

My Notes:

Detail

Keep your heels together
as you perform the roll-up.

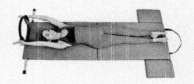

a.

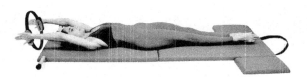

b.

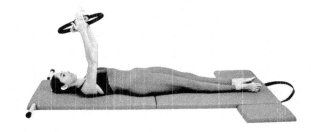

c.

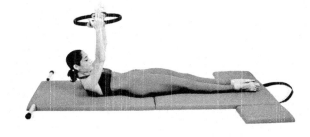

d.

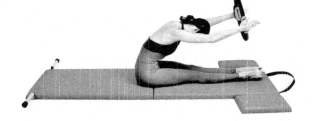

e.

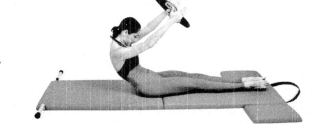

Magic Circle Single Leg Circles

General Purpose:
The single leg circles develop stability in the torso while moving the leg at the hip.

Set-up:
Lift one leg up in the air in Pilates stance, place the cushioned part of the circle over your foot and gently pull down on the circle to stretch the back of your leg for three counts.

Repetitions:
5 circles and reverse with each leg.

Reminder:
Keep your hip anchored to the mat as you stretch your leg (magic circle on your foot). Place the circle between the palms of your hands with your arms extended up towards the sky. Keep constant pressure on the magic circle as you circle your leg.

My Notes:

Stretch your working leg prior to performing the leg circles.

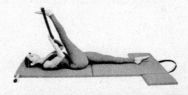

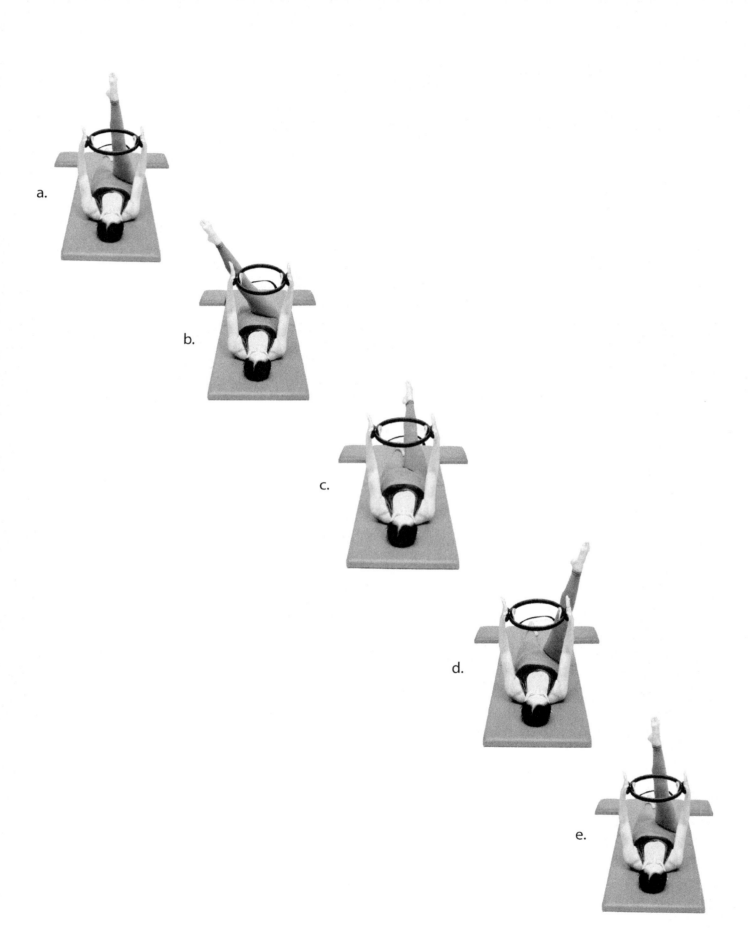

a.

b.

c.

d.

e.

Magic Circle
Rolling Like a Ball

General Purpose:
Rolling like a ball improves balance control and powerhouse strength, and massages the pressure points along both sides of the spine.

Set-up:
Sit up carefully and place your hands on the mat by your hips. With your weight distributed between your hands and feet, lift your seat forward towards the front end of the mat. Place the circle on the inside of your ankles with your hands on the outside of your ankles and your chin towards your chest.

Repetitions:
6 times.

Reminder:
Angle the circle so that it touches your seat. Using the circle for rolling like a ball is a great way to find out if you are kicking your feet away from your seat for momentum. The circle should stay in contact with your seat throughout the rolling movement.

My Notes:

a.

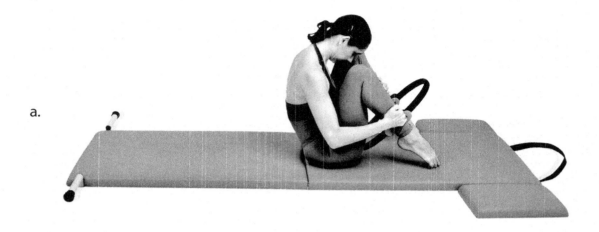

b.

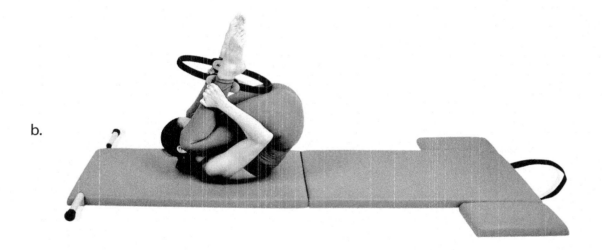

Magic Circle Double Leg Stretch

General Purpose:
The double leg stretch strengthens the powerhouse and improves coordination and breathing.

Set-up:
Draw both knees into your chest with the circle between your ankles. Hands will go on the outside of your ankles.

Repetitions:
5 times.

Reminder:
Squeeze the circle when your legs extend and release the pressure as your legs bend.

My Notes:

a.

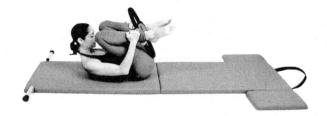

b.

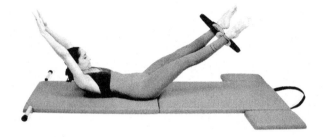

c.

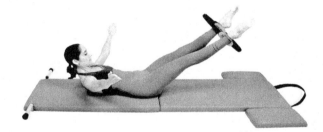

d.

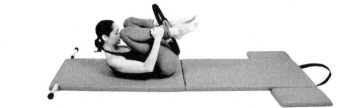

Magic Circle Double Straight Leg

General Purpose:
The double straight leg deepens the powerhouse strength.

Set-up:
Extend both legs up to the sky with the circle between your ankles in Pilates stance and stack your hands behind your head.

Repetitions:
5 times.

Reminder:
Squeeze the circle as you lower your legs (inhale), and release the pressure on the circle as you lift your legs (exhale).

My Notes:

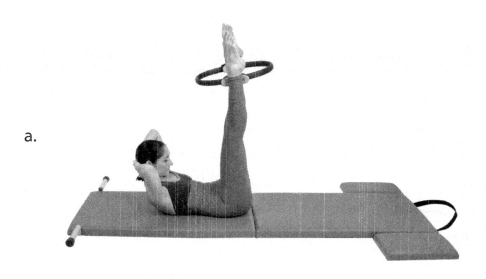

a.

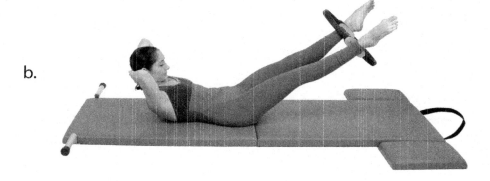

b.

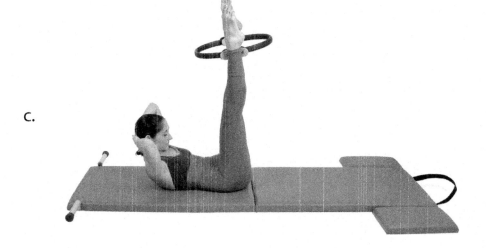

c.

Magic Circle Criss Cross

General Purpose:
The criss cross works the waistline and wrings the air out of the lungs.

Set-up:
Bend both knees to your chest with the circle between your ankles. Keep your hands stacked behind your head with your elbows open wide.

Repetitions:
1-3 sets.

Reminder:
Your legs are bent as you twist from your waist and your legs extend with pressure on the circle on your transition to your other side. If the circle slips out from your ankles on the twist it means you are moving from your hips instead of twisting only from your waist.

My Notes:

a.

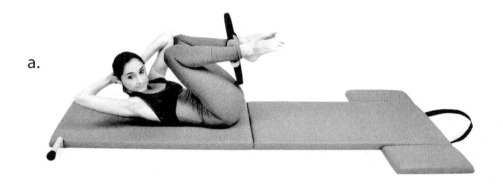

b.

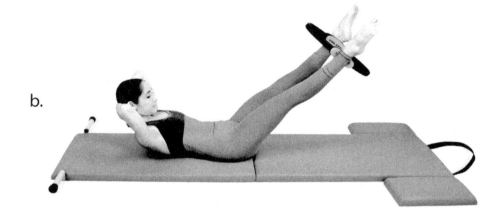

c.

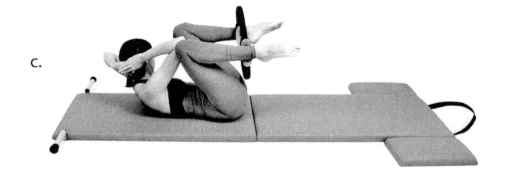

Magic Circle
Single Leg Stretch

General Purpose:
The single leg stretch strengthens the powerhouse and stretches the back.

Set-up:
Place the circle between the palms of your hands. Bend one leg to your chest and extend your other leg out in front of you in Pilates stance.

Repetitions:
6-10 times.

Reminder:
To work your stomach more, keep constant pressure on the circle with long arms (and soft elbows). The focus is on your stomach, not your arms, so avoid the temptation to bend your arms while pressing into the circle.

My Notes:

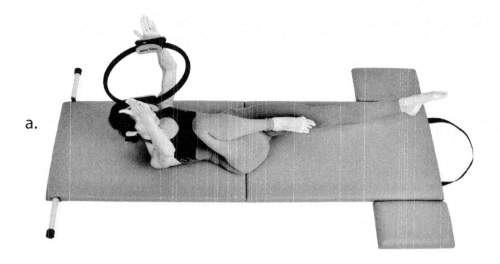

a.

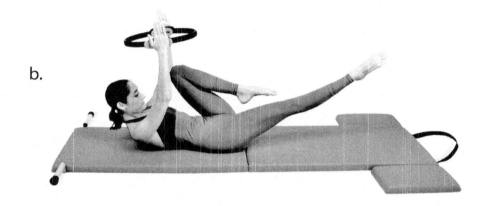

b.

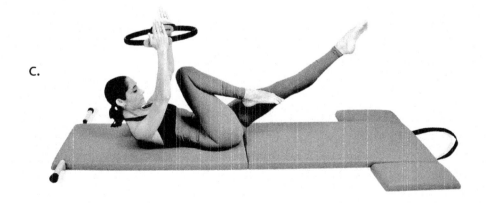

c.

Magic Circle
Single Straight Leg

General Purpose:
The single straight leg strengthens the powerhouse, stretches the back of the raised leg and stretches the front of the hip of the bottom leg.

Set-up:
Extend one leg up towards the sky and extend your other leg out in front of you just a few inches above the mat. Hold the circle between the palms of your hands with your arms extended up towards the sky.

Repetitions:
6-10 times.

Reminder:
Keeping constant pressure on the circle will help stabilize your torso from the movement in your legs.

My Notes:

a.

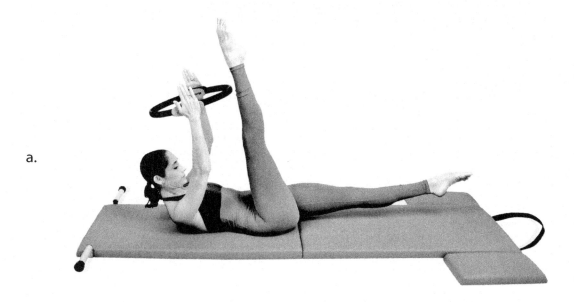

b.

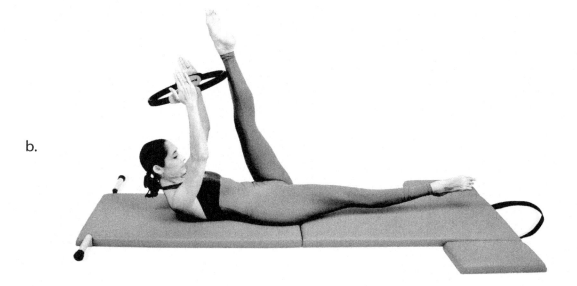

Magic Circle Spine Stretch: Variation One

General Purpose:
The spine stretch forward stretches the spine and the back of the legs, and emphasizes the emptying of the lungs.

Set-up:
Sit up carefully and extend your legs a little wider than your mat and flex your feet. Sit tall with the circle between the palms of your hands. Extend your arms out in front of you at shoulder height.

Repetitions:
3 times.

Reminder:
Press into the circle with long arms as you exhale and bend forward.

My Notes:

a.

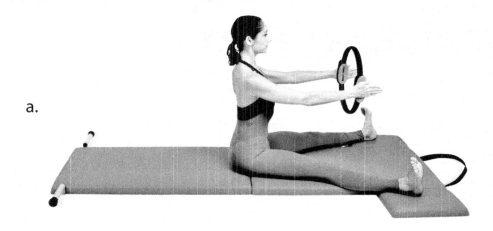

b.

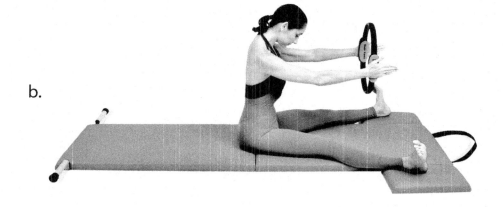

c.

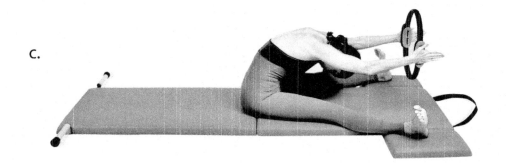

Magic Circle Spine Stretch: Variation Two

General Purpose:
The spine stretch forward stretches the spine and the back of the legs, and emphasizes the emptying of the lungs.

Set-up:
Sit up carefully and extend your legs a little wider than your mat and flex your feet. Place one cushion of the circle on the floor and stack your hands on the top of the other cushion of the circle.

Repetitions:
3 times.

Reminder:
Starting with the bottom cushion of the circle slightly beyond your arm's length distance will give you room to lift through your waistline as you bend forward and press down into the circle. Just be sure to move the top cushion of the circle forward enough so that the circle will be perpendicular to the mat before you press down on it. Keep tension out of your shoulders to keep the work in your powerhouse.

My Notes:

a.

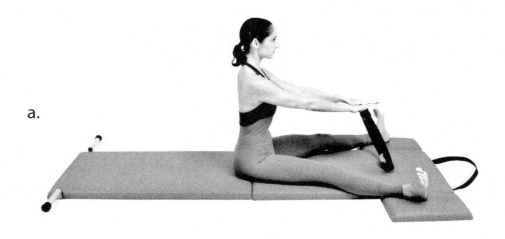

b.

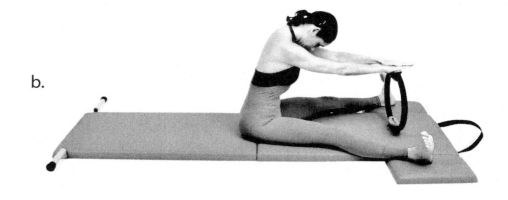

c.

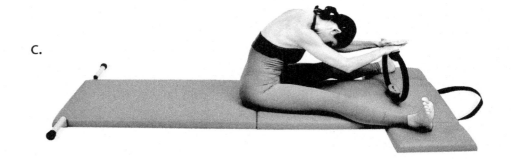

Magic Circle
Open Leg Rocker

General Purpose:
The open leg rocker improves balance control and powerhouse strength, limbers the back of the legs, and massages the pressure points along both sides of the spine.

Set-up:
Bend your legs and place the circle between your ankles. Grab your ankles and extend your legs out in front of you.

Repetitions:
6 times.

Reminder:
Keep pressure on the circle throughout the exercise so that it does not fall. Because your legs are closer together in this version of open leg rocker, you will have to scoop out your abdominals even more to counterbalance the weight of your legs in front of you.

My Notes:

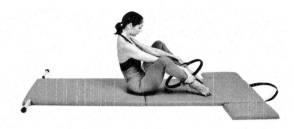

a.

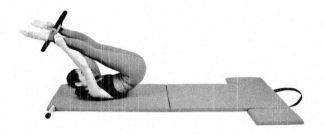

b.

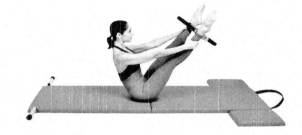

c.

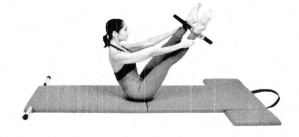

d.

Magic Circle Corkscrew

General Purpose:
The corkscrew strengthens the sides of the body and deepens the powerhouse strength.

Set-up:
With the circle between your ankles, lie down with your arms by your side and your legs extended towards the sky.

Repetitions:
6 times.

Reminder:
Keep constant pressure on the circle as you move your legs. You may have to decrease the circumference of the leg circle movement to counterbalance the weight of the magic circle.

My Notes:

a.

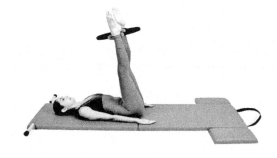

b.

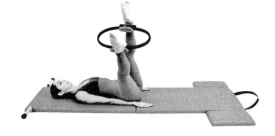

c.

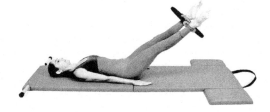

d.

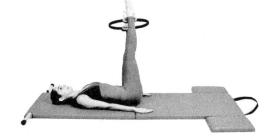

e.

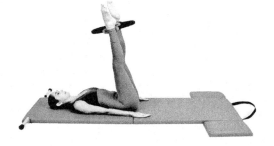

Magic Circle Saw

General Purpose:
The saw works the waistline, wrings the air out of the lungs, opens the lower back, and stretches the back of the legs.

Set-up:
Sit up carefully and extend your legs a little wider than your mat and flex your feet. Sit tall with the circle between the palms of your hands, and extend your arms out in front of you at shoulder height.

Repetitions:
4 times.

Reminder:
Twist tall in your waist and press into the circle as you bend over one of your legs. Be sure to exhale as you press into the circle and keep both hips anchored to the mat.

My Notes:

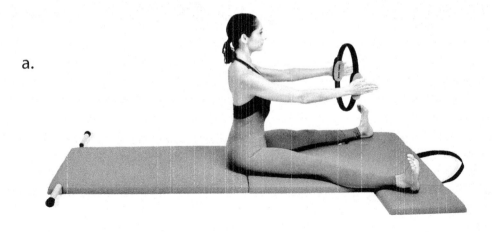

a.

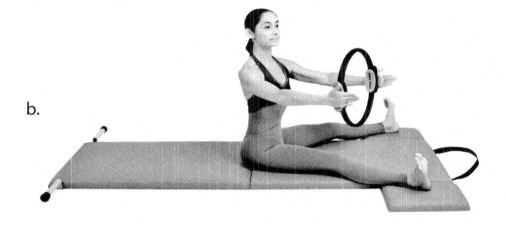

b.

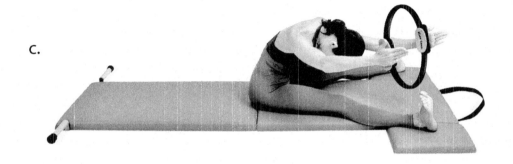

c.

Magic Circle Neck Roll

General Purpose:
The neck roll stretches the neck and opens the chest.

Set-up:
Bring your legs together and turn to your stomach. Prop yourself up on your elbows with the circle flat on the mat between your forearms.

Repetitions:
2 times.

Reminder:
Keep your collar bones open as you press your forearms into the circle.

My Notes:

a.

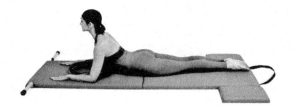

b.

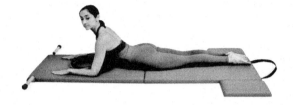

c.

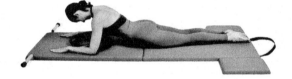

d.

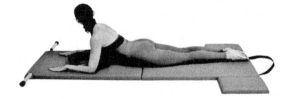

e.

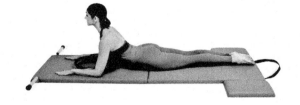

Magic Circle Single Leg Kicks

General Purpose:
The single leg kicks stretch the front of the hips and the top of the thighs while strengthening the seat and back of the legs.

Set-up:
While lying on your stomach with the circle flat on the mat between your forearms, make fists and curl your wrists towards the circle. Your knuckles will not touch each other.

Repetitions:
10 times.

Reminder:
Lift your belly button away from the mat as you press your forearms into the circle.

My Notes:

a.

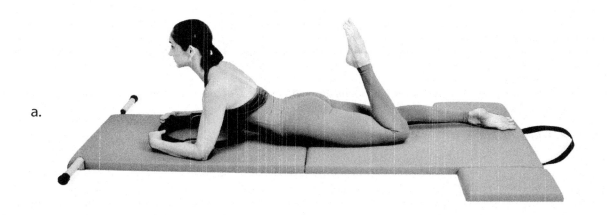

b.

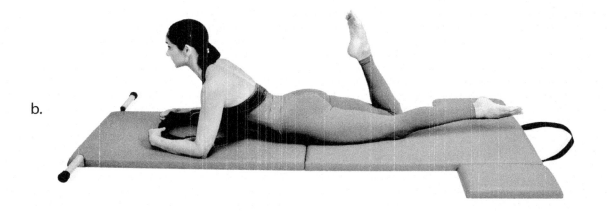

Magic Circle Double Leg Kicks

General Purpose:
The double leg kicks strengthen the back of the legs and open the chest and shoulders.

Set-up:
Place the circle on your back with your hands on the cushions of the circle. Turn your head to one side and rest it on the mat.

Repetitions:
4 times.

Reminder:
Keep the circle on your back as you pulse your heels to your seat 3 times. Extend your arms and legs simultaneously as you lift your chest. The focus is on opening your chest, so do not expect to make the circle move as you press into it with long arms.

My Notes:

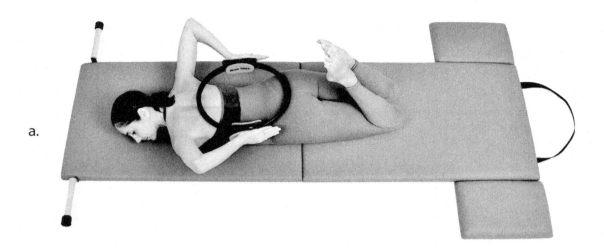

a.

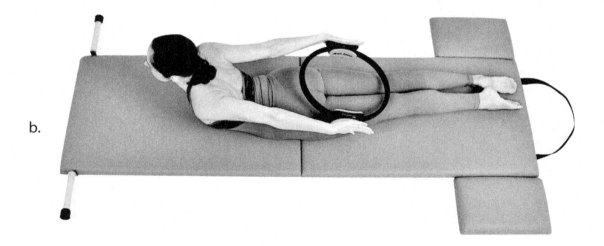

b.

Magic Circle Neck Pull: Variation One

General Purpose:
The neck pull deepens the powerhouse strength and develops articulation of the spine.

Set-up:
Place the circle flat on the mat between your heels. Carefully lie down with your hands stacked behind your head and your elbows wide. Keep your legs parallel with flexed feet.

Repetitions:
3-5 times.

Reminder:
Squeeze the circle without letting it lift off the mat to really work your inner thighs and bottom.

My Notes:

a.

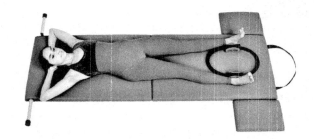

b.

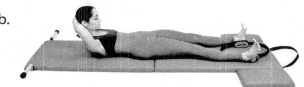

c.

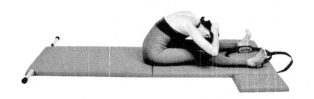

d.

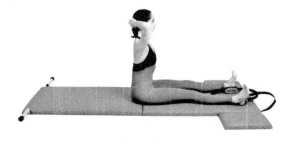

e.

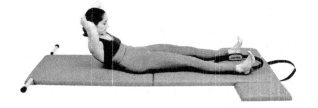

f.

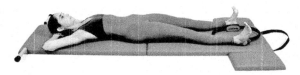

Magic Circle Neck Pull: Variaton Two

General Purpose:
The neck pull deepens the powerhouse strength and develops articulation of the spine.

Set-up:
Stretch your arms up and slightly back with the circle between the palms of your hands. If your back can stay anchored to the mat, place the edge of your circle on the mat behind you. Legs are hip width apart, parallel, with flexed feet.

Repetitions:
3-5 times.

Reminder:
Like the neck pull with the hands stacked behind your head, try to keep your elbows in line with your ears throughout the exercise. For an added challenge, hinge with a flat back (photo E) prior to rolling down onto the mat.

My Notes:

a.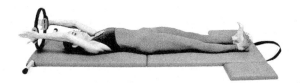

b.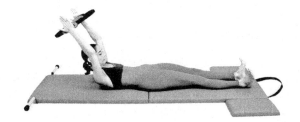

c.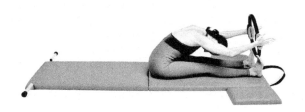

d.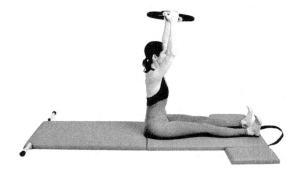

e.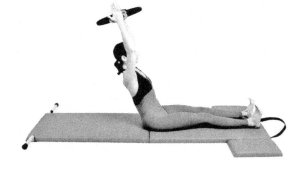

f.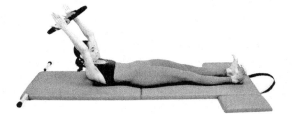

Magic Circle Side Legs: Outer Thighs

General Purpose:
This side leg variation develops torso control and strengthens the outer thighs.

Set-up:
Turn to one side and line your elbow, shoulder, waist and hip with the back edge of the mat. Position both of your feet inside the circle with long legs in front of you and rest your feet off the edge of the mat. Prop your head up with your hand, place your other hand on the mat in front of your waist and keep your gaze straight ahead.

Repetitions:
Press up into the circle with your top leg (as the bottom leg keeps the circle down on the mat) and hold three counts for 3 repetitions. Pulse 5 times.

Reminder:
Lengthen your top leg out from your hip before you press up into the circle.

My Notes:

a.

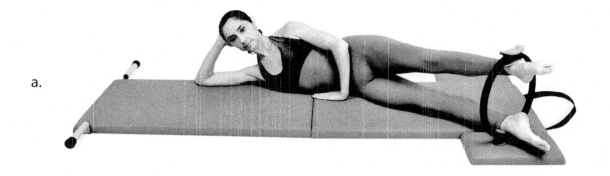

b.

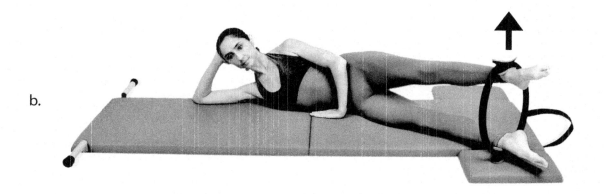

Magic Circle Side Legs: Inner Thighs

General Purpose:
This side leg variation develops torso control and strengthens the inner thighs.

Set-up:
Stay on your side with your elbow, shoulder, waist and hip lined up with the back edge of the mat. With both feet inside the circle, take your top leg out of the circle and place it on top of the cushion of the circle.

Repetitions:
Press down with your top leg and hold three counts for 3 repetitions. Pulse 5 times.

Reminder:
Squeeze your seat to keep the circle steady as you press down on it.

My Notes:

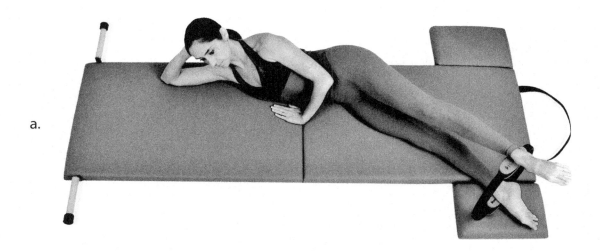

a.

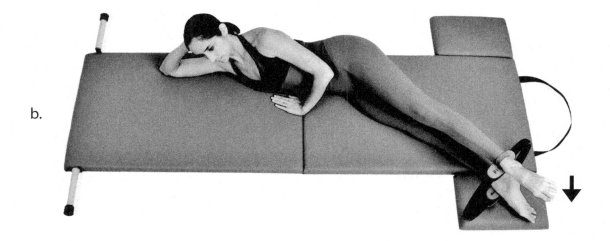

b.

Magic Circle Side Legs: Leg Lifts

General Purpose:
This side leg variation develops torso control and tones the legs.

Set-up:
Stay on your side with your elbow, shoulder, waist and hip lined up with the back edge of the mat. With your bottom foot inside the circle and your top foot outside the circle, tilt the circle back on the edge of the bottom cushion. Take your bottom foot out from the inside of the circle and place it underneath the circle. Stack the cushions of the circle over one another. The circle should be between your ankles.

Repetitions:
Lift your legs while squeezing the circle and hold three counts for 3 repetitions.

Reminder:
For an extra challenge, after the double leg lifts, pulse the circle with your bottom leg only while keeping the circle off the mat (single leg lifts). Next, pulse the circle with both legs while keeping the circle off the mat (leg beats).

My Notes:

Detail

Tilt the circle back on the edge of the bottom cushion to reposition your legs on the circle.

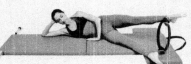

For an added challenge place both hands behind your head.

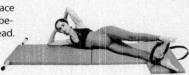

a.

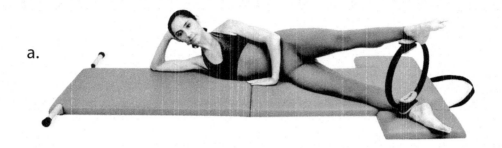

b.

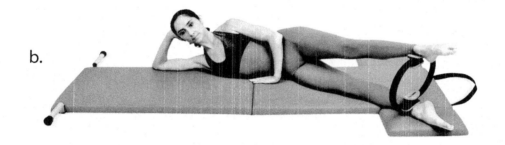

c.

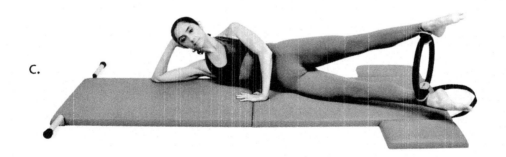

Magic Circle Heel Beats

General Purpose:
The heel beats strengthen the seat and back of the legs, and provide an efficient transition into the side leg series on the other side.

Set-up:
Turn to your stomach and rest your forehead on your hands with the circle between your ankles.

Repetitions:
3 sets of ten beats.

Reminder:
For an added challenge bend your legs and squeeze the circle. Next, keep your legs bent and try to lift your knees and thighs off the mat while squeezing the circle. Be sure to engage your stomach muscles.

My Notes:

Heel Beats

a.

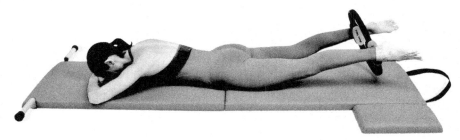

Added Challenge

b.

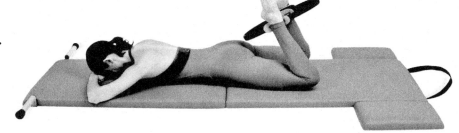

c.

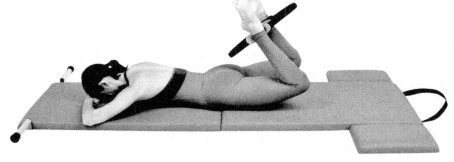

Magic Circle Teaser: Variation One

General Purpose:
The teaser deepens the powerhouse strength, develops articulation of the spine, and works the balance control.

Set-up:
Lie down on your back and draw your knees into your chest. Place the circle between your ankles, and extend your legs forward into the air in a Pilates stance. Extend you arms straight back above the mat in the opposite direction of your legs. Be sure your back is anchored to the mat through your stomach.

Repetitions:
3 times.

Reminder:
Squeeze the circle with your inner thighs to keep the work in your powerhouse. Place your hands behind your legs if you anticipate using your arms for momentum.

My Notes:

a.

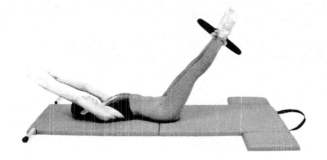

b.

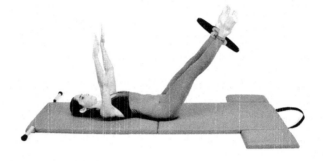

c.

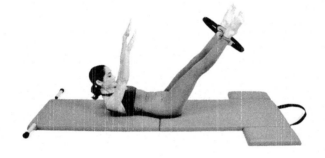

d.

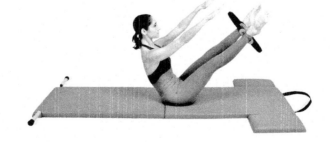

Magic Circle Teaser: Variation Two

General Purpose:
The teaser deepens the powerhouse strength, develops articulation of the spine, and works the balance control.

Set-up:
Lie down on your back and draw your knees into your chest. Place the circle between the palms of your hands and extend your arms straight back above the mat as your legs extend forward into the air in a Pilates stance. Be sure your back is anchored to the mat through your stomach.

Repetitions:
3 times.

Reminder:
As you squeeze the circle with long arms, be sure to keep your shoulders relaxed and your elbows soft.

My Notes:

a.

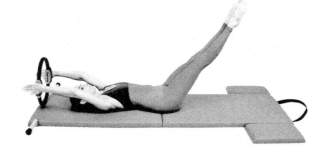

b.

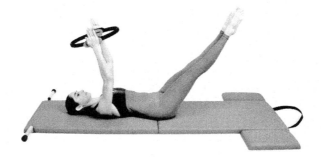

c.

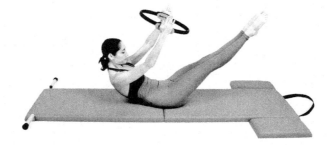

d.

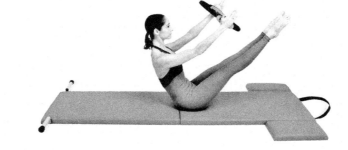

Magic Circle Seal

General Purpose:
The seal is a cool down exercise that improves balance control and powerhouse strength, massages the pressure points along both sides of the spine, and develops coordination.

Set-up:
Sit up carefully and place the circle between your ankles with your arms interlaced through your legs.

Repetitions:
6 times.

Reminder:
Your insteps will not click as you use your inner thighs to pulse the circle. Remember to work your inner thighs with the same intensity when you perform the seal without the circle.

My Notes:

a.

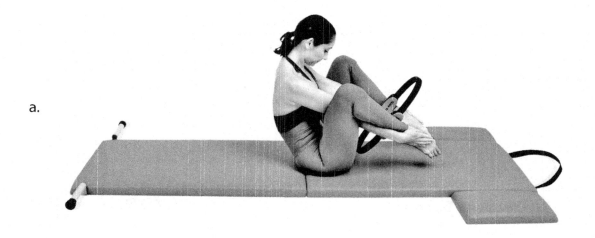

b.

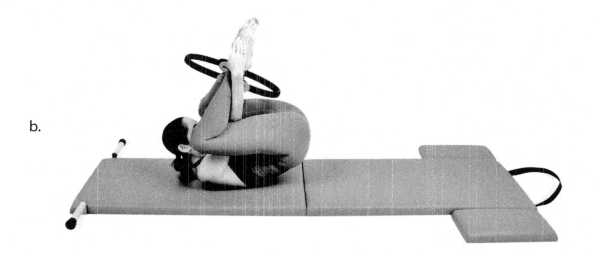

The Standing Weights Series

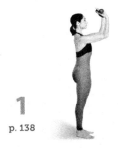

1
p. 138

90 Degrees Forward

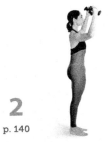

2
p. 140

90 Degrees Side

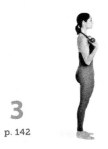

3
p. 142

Standing Curls

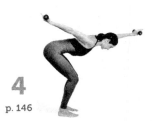

4
p. 146

Boxing

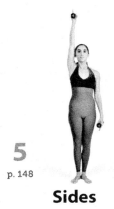

5
p. 148

Sides

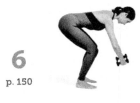

6
p. 150

Bug

The standing weights series is composed of three different postures of varying degrees of difficulty. Exercises performed standing vertical are basic to basic-intermediate level, the table top exercises are intermediate level, and the lunges are intermediate-advanced level.

Perform the series in the sequence shown here. If you come to an exercise that you have not learned in the studio with your instructor, skip it, and go to the next familiar exercise in the series.

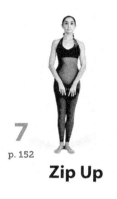

7
p. 152

Zip Up

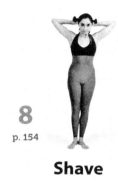

8
p. 154

Shave

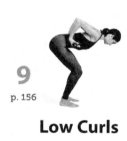

9
p. 156

Low Curls

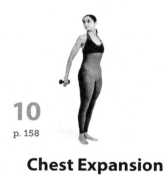

10
p. 158

Chest Expansion

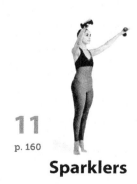

11
p. 160

Sparklers

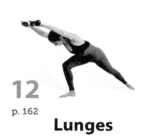

12
p. 162

Lunges

90 Degrees Arms Forward

General Purpose:
The 90 degrees arms forward exercise strengthens the top of the upper arms and the shoulders.

Set-up:
Stand in Pilates stance with your arms bent in front of you at a 90 degree angle.

Repetitions:
3-5 times.

Reminder:
Since you should <u>create resistance</u> with every movement, weights are not necessary for these exercises. If you do use them, always hold the weights with long fingers and use no more than 3 pound weights in each hand.

My Notes:

Take your finger tips towards your shoulders for an added challenge.

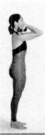

a.

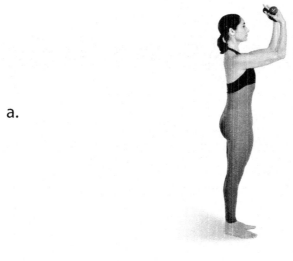

b.

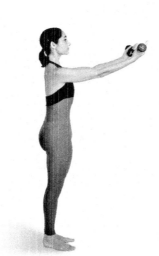

c.

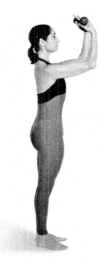

90 Degrees Arms Side

General Purpose:
The 90 degrees arms side exercise strengthens the top of the upper arms, the shoulders, and the upper back.

Set-up:
Stand in Pilates stance with your arms to the side bent at a 90 degree angle.

Repetitions:
3-5 times.

Reminder:
Avoid dropping your elbows as you extend your arms.

My Notes:

Detail

Take your finger tips towards your shoulders for an added challenge.

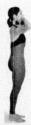

a.

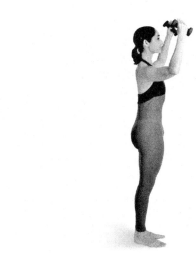

b.

c.

Standing Curls

General Purpose:
The standing curls exercise strengthens the top of the upper arms and the forearms.

Set-up:
Stand in Pilates stance with your arms long by your sides, your palms facing forward.

Repetitions:
3-5 times.

Reminder:
Each arm curl is followed by an extension of your arms and can finish with flexion in your wrists.

My Notes:

a.

b.

c.

d.

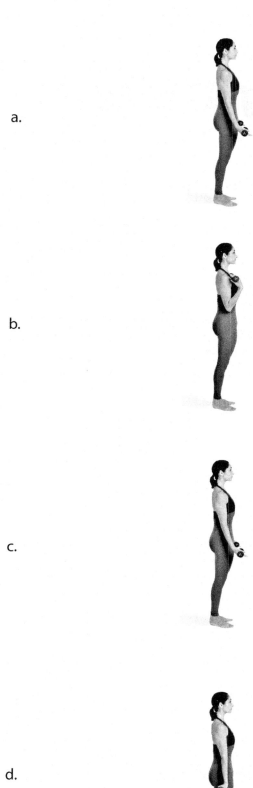

Standing Triceps

General Purpose:
The standing triceps exercise strengthens the back of the upper arms and upper back, and opens the chest.

Set-up:
Stand in Pilates stance with your arms bent and your elbows pointed behind you. Position your hands near your waist with your palms facing up.

Repetitions:
3-5 times.

Reminder:
After your arms extend behind you, try to squeeze them towards one another as if hiding them behind your back. If the table top position is available to you, you can skip this exercise and do the table top version of the triceps later on in the series. (See Low Curls.)

My Notes:

a.

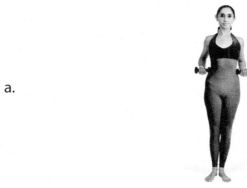

b.

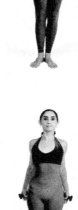

c.

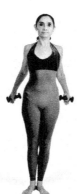

d.

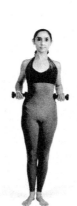

Boxing

General Purpose:
The boxing exercise strengthens the back of the arms, legs, and shoulders, and develops strength and stabilization in the torso.

Set-up:
From a standing Pilates stance position, separate your heels so that you are standing in parallel with your heels hip width apart. Bend your arms at your elbows with the palms of your hands facing forward. Start to bend your legs as you maintain a lift through your powerhouse. Keeping your legs bent, hinge at your hips with a flat back into your table top position.

Repetitions:
3 sets.

Reminder:
In the table top position, keep your knees bent over your toes with your stomach pulled in. Your shoulders should remain still as your arms pass each other.

My Notes:

Detail

Transition into boxing

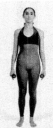

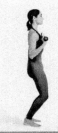

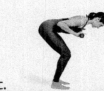

a.   b.   c.

a.

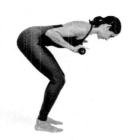

b.

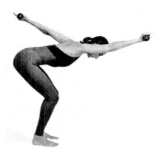

c.

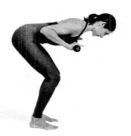

d.

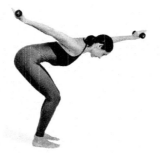

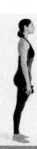

Sides

General Purpose:
This exercise stretches and strengthens the sides of the body.

Set-up:
Stand in Pilates stance with one arm extended towards the sky and pressed towards your ear. Your other arm should hang by your side.

Repetitions:
4 times.

Reminder:
Keep your arm pressed to your ear as you come out of the side bend to really work your sides.

My Notes:

Detail

Keep your elbows within the frame of your body in your transition to the other side.

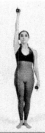

a.

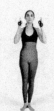

b.

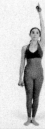

c.

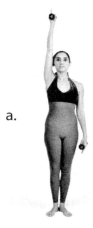

a.

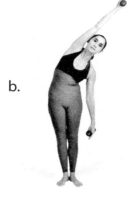

b.

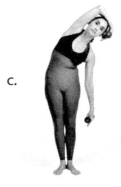

c.

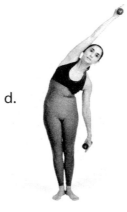

d.

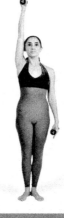

e.

Bug

General Purpose:
The bug exercise strengthens arms, legs and upper back, opens the chest, and develops strength and stabilization in the torso.

Set-up:
From a standing Pilates stance position, separate your heels so that you are standing in parallel with your heels hip width apart. Extend your arms forward with your palms facing each other, and have a slight bend in your elbows. Start to bend your legs as you maintain a lift through your powerhouse. Keeping your legs bent, hinge at your hips with a flat back into your table top position.

Repetitions:
3-5 times.

Reminder:
Keep the back of your neck long in your table top position.

My Notes:

Detail

Transition into the bug

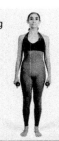

a.

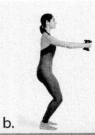

b.

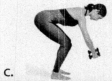

c.

a.

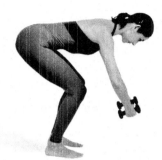

b.

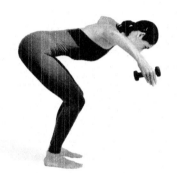

c.

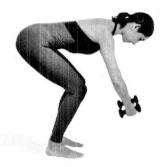

Transition out of the bug

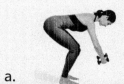

a.

b.

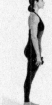

c.

Zip Up

General Purpose:
The zip up exercise strengthens the shoulders, arms, and sides of the body.

Set-up:
Stand in Pilates stance with your arms long in front of your legs and your hand weights together.

Repetitions:
3-5 times.

Reminder:
Be sure to coordinate the lift of your powerhouse with the lift of your arms. Your elbows should stay lower than your shoulders when lifting the weights. For an added challenge, rise onto your half toe with your heels glued together as you "zip" the weights up the center of your body.

My Notes:.

a.

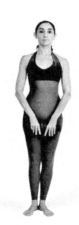

b.

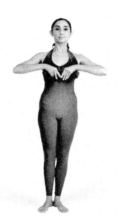

c.

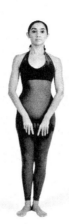

Shave

General Purpose:
The shave exercise opens the chest and shoulders, and strengthens the arms and upper back.

Set-up:
Stand in Pilates stance with your arms long in front of your legs and weights together. Start to lift the weights up the center of your body and over your head with your elbows open. Keep your gaze straight ahead.

Repetitions:
3-5 times.

Reminder:
If starting the shave with the weights at the base of your skull is not available to you, try beginning the movement with the weights in front of your forehead (salute position). For an added challenge, rise onto your half toe with your heels glued together as you "shave" the back of your head.

My Notes:

Transition into shave

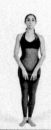

a.

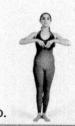

b.

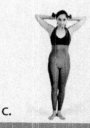

c.

a.

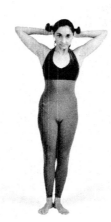

b.

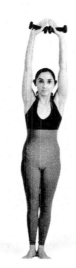

c.

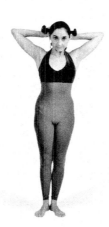

Low Curls

General Purpose:
The low curls strengthen the back of the arms, legs and upper back, opens the chest, and develops strength and stabilization in the torso.

Set-up:
From a standing Pilates stance position, separate your heels so that you are standing in parallel with your heels hip width apart. Bend your arms with your elbows by your sides and your fingers pointed towards your shoulders (your palms will be facing you). Start to bend your legs as you maintain a lift through your powerhouse. Keeping your legs bent, hinge at your hips with a flat back into your table top position.

Repetitions:
3-5 times.

Reminder:
For an added challenge, progress to curls with the elbows starting above your table top position.

My Notes:

Transition into low curls

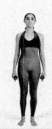

a.

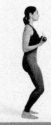

b.

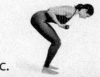

c.

Low Curls

a.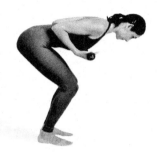

b.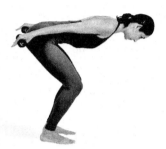

Added Challenge

c.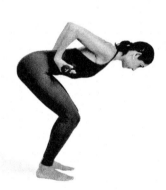

d.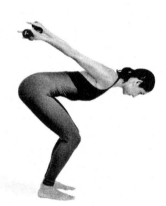

Transition out of low curls

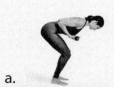

a.

b.

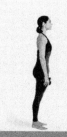

c.

Chest Expansion

General Purpose:
The chest expansion is a breathing exercise that opens the chest, stretches the neck, and strengthens the ocular muscles.

Set-up:
Stand in Pilates stance with your arms extended in front of you at shoulder width apart.

Repetitions:
4 times.

Reminder:
Isolate your shoulders as you turn your head.

My Notes:

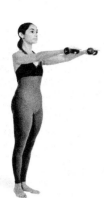

a.

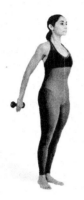

b.

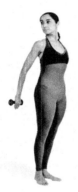

c.

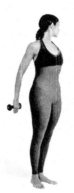

d.

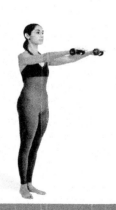

e.

Sparklers

General Purpose:
The sparklers exercise strengthens the upper arms and shoulders, and develops torso control.

Set-up:
Stand in Pilates stance with your arms long in front of you.

Repetitions:
2-3 sets.

Reminder:
As your arms lift and simultaneously draw little circles in the air, avoid the temptation to shift your weight back into your heels. For an added challenge, rise onto your half toe as your arms circle upwards, then slowly lower your heels as your arms reverse the circles on the way down.

My Notes:

a.

b.

c.

d.

e.

f.

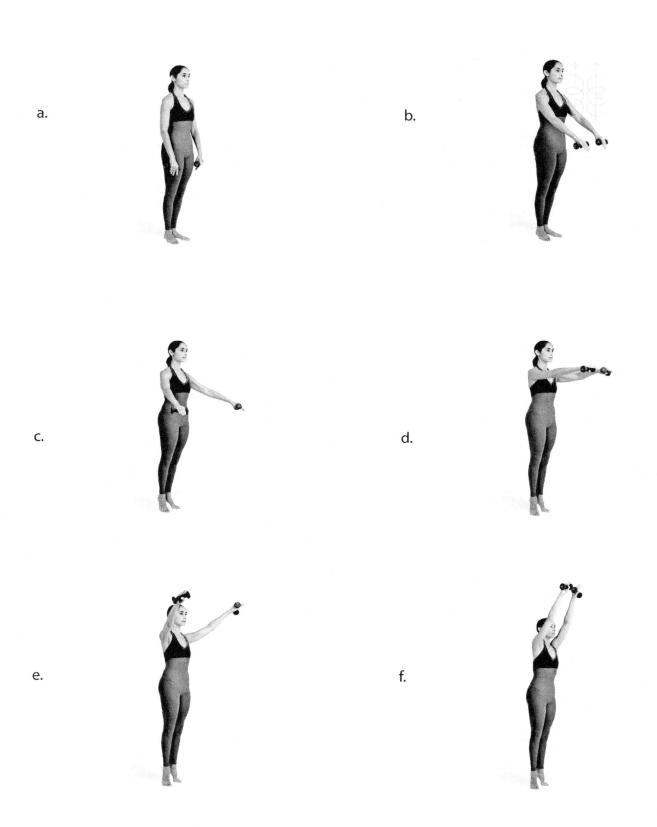

Lunges

General Purpose:
The lunges strengthen the legs, arms, back and shoulders, and develop strength and stability in the torso.

Set-up:
Stand in Pilates stance and move one heel slightly in front of the instep of your other foot. Turn your hips and shoulders to the direction in which the toes of your front foot are pointing. Slide your front foot out on a forward diagonal and lunge forward with your knee over your toes and your arms extended long in front of you.

Repetitions:
3- 5 arm lifts on each side.

Reminder:
Keep your front leg at a 90 degree angle, and keep your waist lifted above your thigh in the lunge.

My Notes:

a.

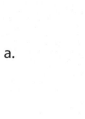

b.

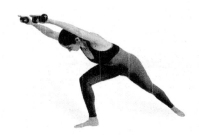

c.

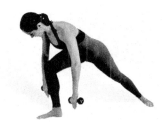

d.

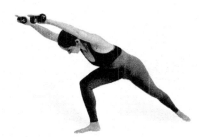

The Magic Circle Exercises

1

p. 166-167

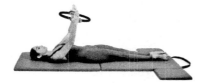

Arm Exercises Lying Down

2

p. 168-169

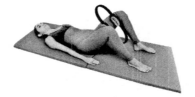

Leg Exercises Lying Down

3

p. 170-175

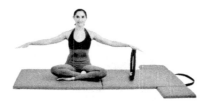

Exercises Seated On Mat

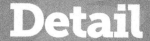

Detail

Unlike all the other chapters in this book, the exercises represented in this chapter do not need to be performed as an entire series. You can pick the exercises that best suit your needs.

4
p. 176-179

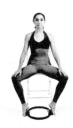

Chair Exercises

5
p. 180-185

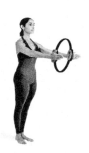

Arm Exercises Standing

6
p. 186-189

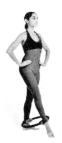

Leg Exercises Standing

7
p. 190-195

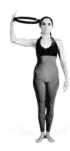

Neck Exercises

Arm Exercises Lying Down

General Purpose:
The arm exercises lying down strengthen the arms while providing back support.

Set-up:
Lie down with your legs extended on the mat in Pilates stance. Place the circle between the palms of your hands and extend your arms up towards the sky.

Repetitions:
Press into the circle and hold for 3 counts in each position for 3 repetitions (start with your arms straight up towards the sky, then lower your arms down towards your legs, and finish with your arms reaching up and slightly behind you). To complete the series, lower your arms down towards your legs and begin to pulse into the circle with long arms as you lift them up towards the sky and slightly behind you. Continue to pulse into the circle as you lower your arms back down towards your legs. Repeat the movement for 2 more sets.

Reminder:
Keep the circle between the palms of your hands with long arms, fingers extended and soft elbows. If it is hard to keep your spine anchored to the mat, you can bend your legs slightly with your feet remaining on the mat.

My Notes:

a.

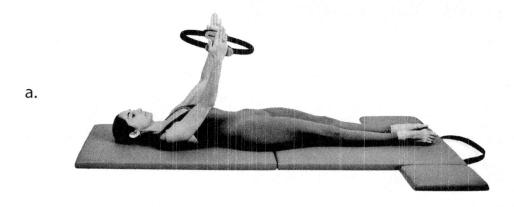

b.

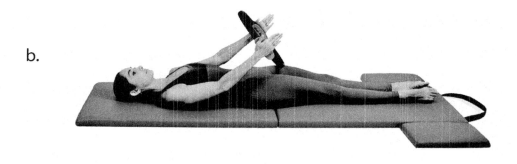

c.

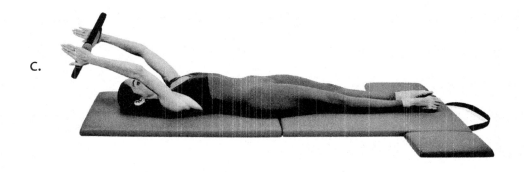

Leg Exercises Lying Down

General Purpose:
The leg exercises lying down strengthen the inner thighs while providing back support.

Set-up:
Lie down with your legs bent and your feet parallel apart on the mat. Place the circle between your inner thighs.

Repetitions:
Press into the circle and hold 3 counts for 3-5 repetitions.

Reminder:
For an added challenge, you can repeat the sequence with your hips in the air.

My Notes:

Basic Variation

a.

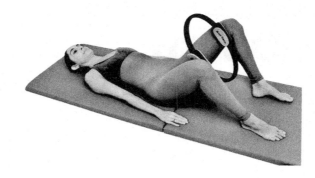

b.

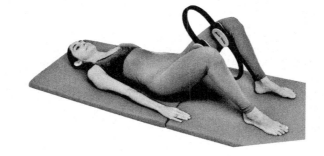

Added Challenge

c.

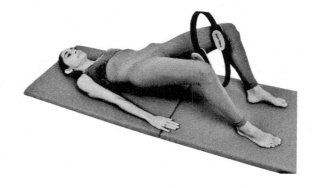

d.

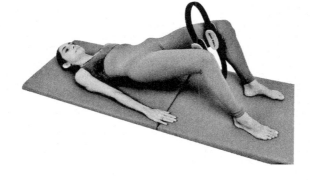

Seated On Mat: Roll Down

General Purpose:
The roll down strengthens the powerhouse and develops articulation of the spine.

Set-up:
Sit with your legs bent and your feet parallel apart on the mat. Place the circle between your inner thighs, and position your hands lightly behind your thighs.

Repetitions:
3-5 times.

Reminder:
Be sure to keep the circle between your inner thighs. If it slides up to your knees, stop, and re-position the circle.

My Notes:

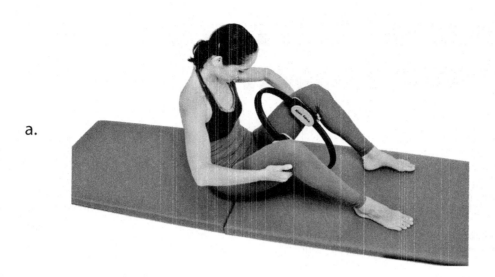

a.

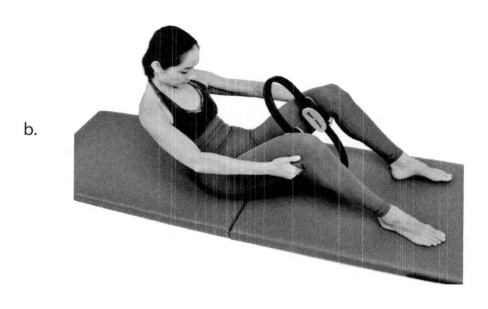

b.

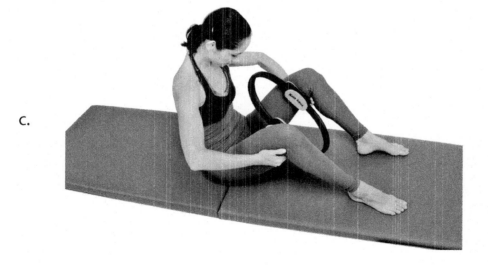

c.

Seated On Mat: Press Down

General Purpose:
The press down exercise strengthens the under arms, develops shoulder control, and improves posture.

Set-up:
Sit with bent legs crossed and position the circle perpendicular to the mat under the palm of your hand.

Repetitions:
Press down and hold 3 counts for 3 repetitions on each side.

Reminder:
Maintain the evenness in your hips and shoulders as you press down on the circle.

My Notes:

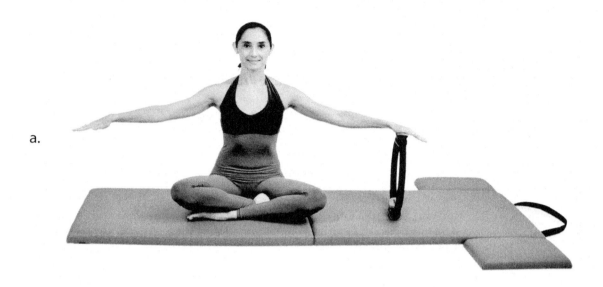

a.

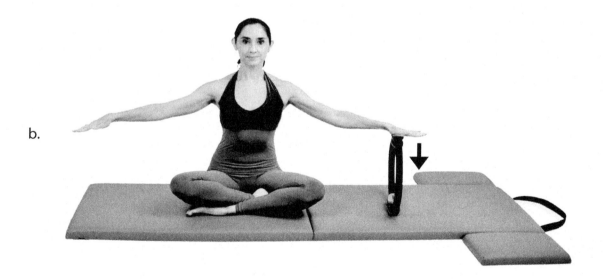

b.

Seated On Mat: Mermaid/King of Neptune

General Purpose:
The mermaid/king of Neptune exercise strengthens the under arms, develops shoulder control, and stretches the sides of the body.

Set-up:
Sit with bent legs crossed and place the circle on the mat a little beyond your arm's length.

Repetitions:
Press down and hold 3 counts for 3 repetitions on each side.

Reminder:
Lift your powerhouse and start to bend your torso towards the circle. Be sure to move the top cushion of the circle so that the circle is perpendicular to the mat before you press down on it. Try to keep your raised arm pressed to your ear throughout the exercise.

My Notes:

a.

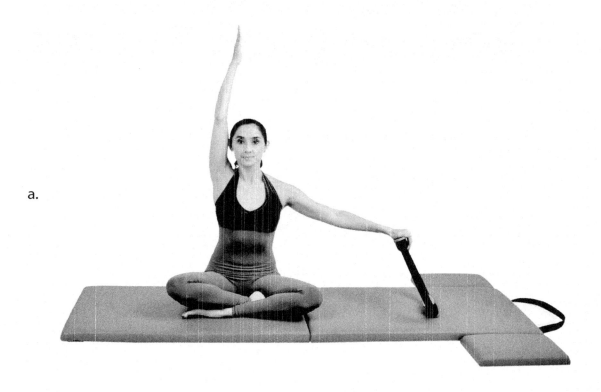

b.

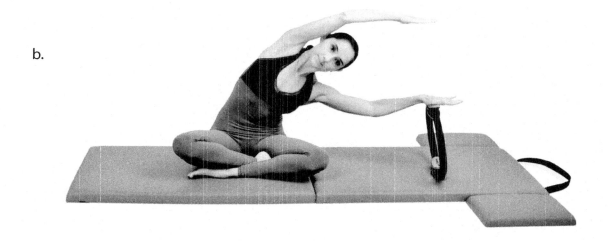

Chair Exercise: Circle Between Inner Thighs

General Purpose:
The seated exercise with the circle between the legs strengthens the seat and inner thighs, and improves the posture.

Set-up:
Sit at the front edge of a chair with your feet on the floor, parallel apart. Place the circle between your inner thighs.

Repetitions:
Press in and hold 3 counts for 3-5 repetitions.

Reminder:
Be sure to squeeze your seat in addition to working your inner thighs.

My Notes:

a.

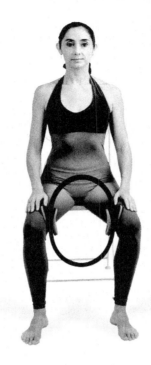

b.

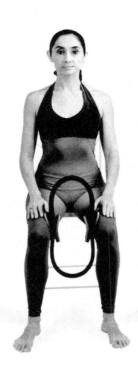

Chair Exercise: Circle Between Feet

General Purpose:
The seated exercise with the circle between the feet strengthens the back of the legs, seat, and inner thighs.

Set-up:
Sit at the front edge of a chair with the circle flat on the floor and the soles of your feet on the circle.

Repetitions:
Press in and hold 3 counts for 3-5 repetitions.

Reminder:
Be sure to press your feet into the circle with equal amounts of pressure.

My Notes:

a.

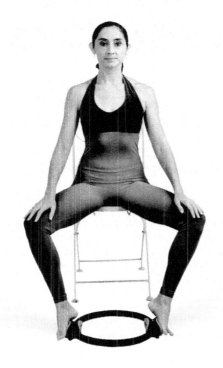

b.

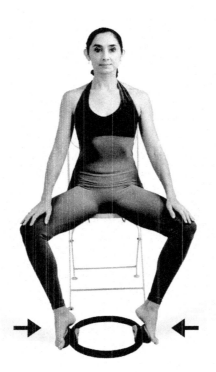

Arm Exercises Standing: Arms Forward

General Purpose:
The arms forward exercise improves posture and tones the arms.

Set-up:
Stand in Pilates stance with the circle between the palms of your hands. Extend your arms forward to your waist level.

Repetitions:
Press into the circle and hold for 3 counts in each position for 3 repetitions (start with your arms at waist level, then lower your arms down towards your legs, and finish with your arms up towards the sky). To complete the series, lower your arms down towards your legs and begin to pulse into the circle with long arms as you lift them up in front of you and towards the sky. Continue to pulse into the circle as you lower your arms back down towards your legs. Repeat the movement for 2 more sets.

Reminder:
Lift your belly button in and up before you press into the circle. For an added challenge, you can rise up onto your half toe as your arms pulse upwards, and slowly lower your heels as your arms pulse down towards your legs.

My Notes:

Part One

a.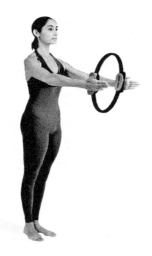

b.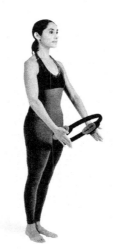

c.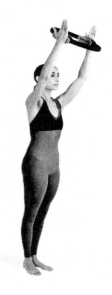

Part Two

a.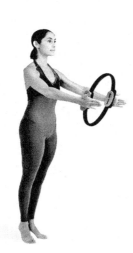

b.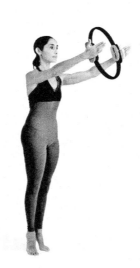

c.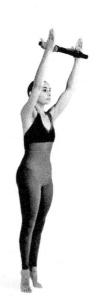

Arm Exercises Standing: Side Arm

General Purpose:
The side arm exercise strengthens the under arms, the sides of the body, and the upper back.

Set-up:
Standing in Pilates stance, hold one cushion of the circle and place the other cushion of the circle on the side of your body, just under your hip bone. Keep the elbow of your working arm slightly lifted.

Repetitions:
Press in and hold 3 counts for 3-5 repetitions on each side.

Reminder:
If you have a noticeable discrepancy in strength between your two sides, start the sequence with your weaker side, then repeat with your stronger side, and finish with extra sets on your weaker side.

My Notes:

a.

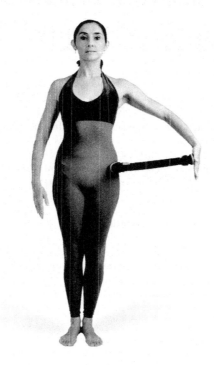

b.

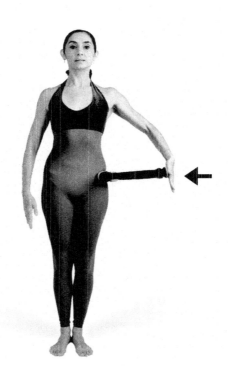

Arm Exercises Standing: Arms Behind Back

General Purpose:
The exercise with the arms behind the back opens the chest, strengthens the upper back, and improves posture.

Set-up:
Stand in Pilates stance with your arms long behind you and the circle between the palms of your hands (finger tips pointing down). The circle will be perpendicular to the floor.

Repetitions:
Press in and hold 3 counts for 3-5 repetitions.

Reminder:
Maintain good posture and long arms when pressing into the circle. Do not expect the circle to move.

My Notes:

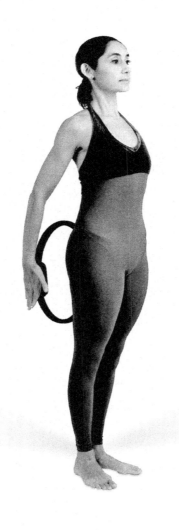

Leg Exercises Standing: Plie (Knee Bends)

General Purpose:
The plie exercise strengthens the inner thighs.

Set-up:
Place the circle just above your ankles and stand with your legs slightly turned out.

Repetitions:
Press in and hold 3 counts for 3-5 repetitions.

Reminder:
Maintain a long line down the front of your hips throughout the exercise (in other words, avoid a backward tilt in your pelvis).

My Notes:

a.

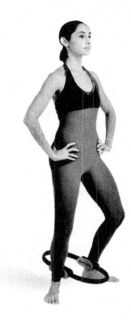

b.

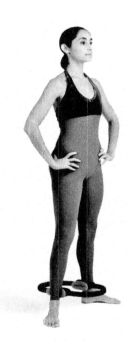

Leg Exercises Standing: Leg Push Down

General Purpose:
The leg push down series develops balance control and strengthens the inner thighs.

Set-up:
Place the circle between your ankles and shift your weight onto one leg with your other leg raised to the side. Place your hands on your hips or extend them out to the side.

Repetitions:
Press into the circle and hold 3 counts for 3 repetitions, then shift onto your other leg and repeat.

Reminder:
Start out shifting your weight from side to side (photos C and D). Later on you may be able to do the variation with your weight shifting from front to back(photos A-B and E-F). For more of a challenge, shift your weight in all directions. An example of the ideal order for the full form is: right leg front, left leg back, right leg side, left leg side, right leg back, left leg front (starting with one leg front, and finishing with your other leg front).

My Notes:

Complete Sequence

a.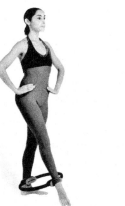

b.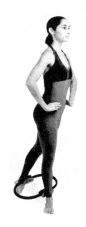

c.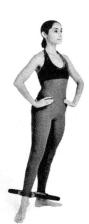

d.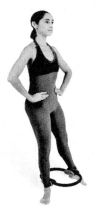

e.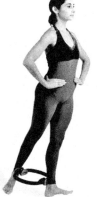

f.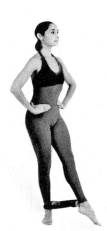

Neck Exercises: Under Chin

General Purpose:
The neck exercise with the circle below the chin stretches the back of the neck.

Set-up:
Stand in Pilates stance with the cushioned part of the circle below your chin and your hands stacked under the bottom cushion of the circle.

Repetitions:
As you lower your chin towards your chest, press your chin into the circle and hold 3 counts for 3 repetitions.

Reminder:
Hold the circle steady as your chin presses into it. Your arms should not drop.

My Notes:

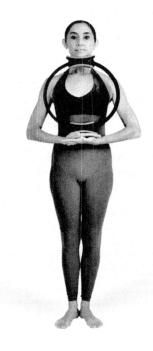

a.

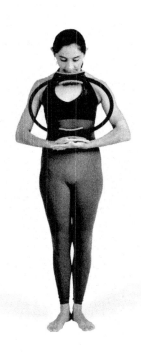

b.

Neck Exercises: Forehead

General Purpose:
The neck exercise with the circle on the forehead strengthens the back of the neck.

Set-up:
Stand in Pilates stance with the cushioned part of the circle on your forehead and your hands stacked in front of the other cushioned part of the circle. The circle should be parallel with the floor.

Repetitions:
Press your hands into the circle and hold 3 counts for 3 repetitions.

Reminder:
Keep your weight light on your heels when pushing the circle back into your forehead (your head should stay stationary). This exercise can also be performed without the circle (stack your hands and place them directly on your forehead).

My Notes:

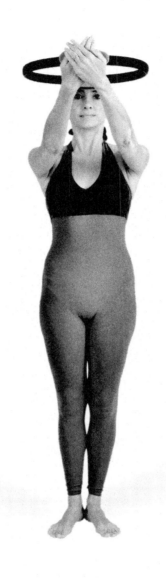

Neck Exercises: Side of Head

General Purpose:
The neck exercise with the circle on the side of the head strengthens the sides of the neck.

Set-up:
Stand in Pilates stance with one hand on the cushion of the circle and the other cushioned part of the circle on the side of your head (just above your ear). The circle will be parallel with the floor.

Repetitions:
Press your hand into the circle and hold 3 counts for 3 repetitions, then repeat to the other side.

Reminder:
Keep your head centered on your body as your hand presses into the circle (your head should stay stationary). This exercise can also be performed without the circle (place the heel of your hand directly on the side of your head).

My Notes:

a.

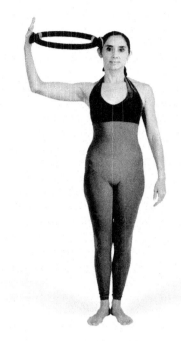

b.

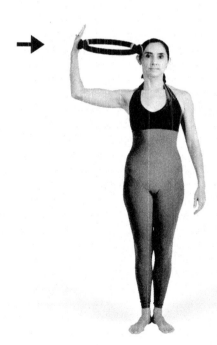

The Wall Series

1
p. 198

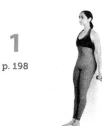

Preparation

2
p. 200

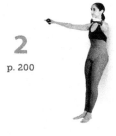

Arm Circles

3
p. 202

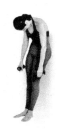

Peel Down

4
p. 204

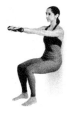

Squats

5
p. 206

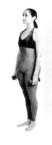

Wall Ending

Wall Preparation

General Purpose:
The wall preparation exercise aligns the body, works the breathing, and opens the chest.

Set-up:
Stand in Pilates stance with the back of your body (including heels) touching the wall. Walk your feet away from the wall and go into Pilates stance as you pull your stomach in and anchor your spine to the wall. With your arms extended in front of you at shoulder height, start to inhale as you lower your arms and press the palms of your hands into the wall, exhale as your arms float forward again.

Repetitions:
3 times.

Reminder:
You may need to keep the back of your head away from the wall to avoid tension in your neck. The wall series can be performed with or without hand weights.

My Notes:

a.

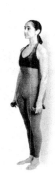

b.

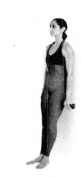

c.

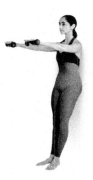

d.

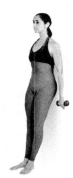

Arm Circles

General Purpose:
The arm circles exercise strengthens the arms and shoulders, develops symmetry of movement in the arms, stabilizes the torso from the movement in the arms, and promotes good posture.

Set-up:
Keep your back anchored to the wall with your feet away from the wall in Pilates stance. Bring the hand weights together in front of your legs and lift your arms up through the center of your body. Open your arms without letting them get past your field of vision and circle your arms down.

Repetitions:
3 circles and reverse.

Reminder:
Be sure to move your arms in a range that does not pull your back away from the wall. Watch for evenness in your arms.

My Notes:

a.

b.

c.

d.

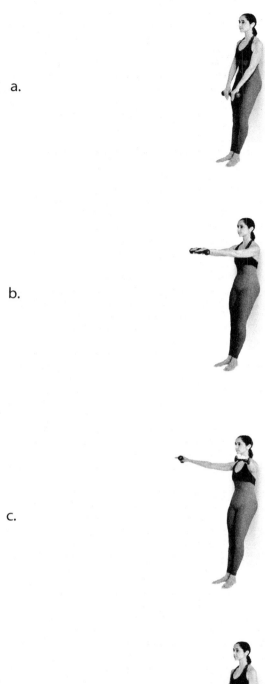

Peel Down

General Purpose:
The peel down develops articulation of the spine, opens the lower back, and empties the lungs.

Set-up:
Keep your back anchored to the wall with your feet away from the wall in Pilates stance. Peel your spine away from the wall deliberately with your stomach engaged.

Repetitions:
2 times.

Reminder:
Lower your head and exhale as you peel your spine off the wall. Breathe naturally as your arms hang. Do five little circles in each direction with your arms hanging. Inhale as you roll your back up the wall.

My Notes:

a.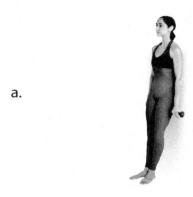

b.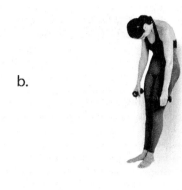

c.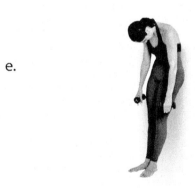

d.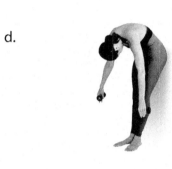

e.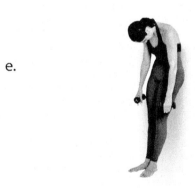

f.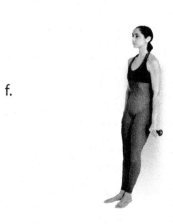

Squats

General Purpose:
The squats strengthen the legs, seat and stomach.

Set-up:
Separate your heels hip width apart parallel and move your feet a little further forward keeping your back against the wall. As your back slides down the wall into your squat, extend your arms out in front of you to a height that still allows you to keep your back pressed into the wall.

Repetitions:
3 times.

Reminder:
Be sure your hips do not go lower than your knee level in the squat.

My Notes:

Detail

For more of a challenge, lift your arms up towards the sky on the squat.

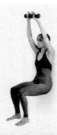

a.

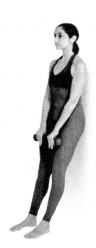

b.

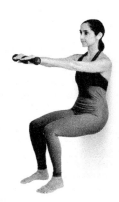

c.

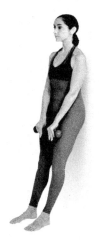

Wall Ending

General Purpose:
The wall ending reiterates the importance of incorporating your Pilates skills into the way you stand and move throughout your day.

Set-up:
Walk your feet back into the wall in Pilates stance. With long arms, press your palms back into the wall and take a few steps forward, bringing your arms down by your side.

Repetitions:
1 time.

Reminder:
Finish standing away from the wall in Pilates stance with your belly button pulled in and up and your weight forward on the balls of your feet.

My Notes:

a.

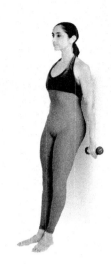

b.

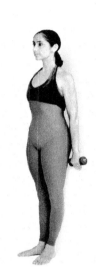

c.

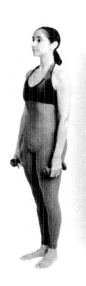

The Basic Reformer

1

p. 216-223

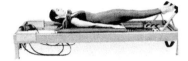

Footwork

2

p. 224

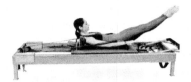

Hundred

3

p. 272-275

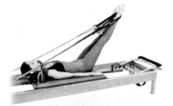

Leg Circles and Frog

4

p. 262

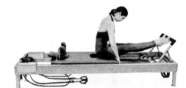

Stomach Massage Round

5

p. 264

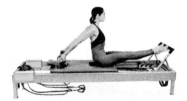

Stomach Massage Hands Back

6

p. 266

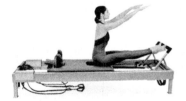

Stomach Massage Reach Up

7

p. 244

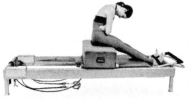

Short Box Round

8

p. 246

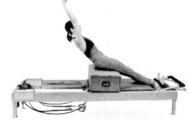

Short Box Flat

Detail

The basic reformer workout introduces various postures on the reformer apparatus in a sequence that flows full circle from lying down, to sitting, standing, kneeling and lying down again.

9
p. 248

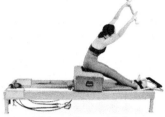

Short Box Side

10
p. 252

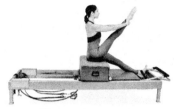

Short Box Tree

11
p. 260

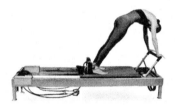

Elephant

12
p. 276

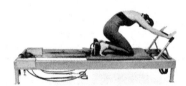

Kneeling Knee Stretches Round

13
p. 278

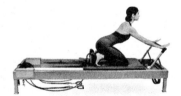

Kneeling Knee Stretches Arched

14
p. 280

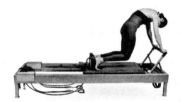

Kneeling Knee Stretches Off

15
p. 282

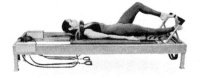

Running

16
p. 284

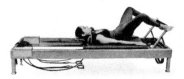

Pelvic Lift

The Intermediate Reformer

1
p. 216-223

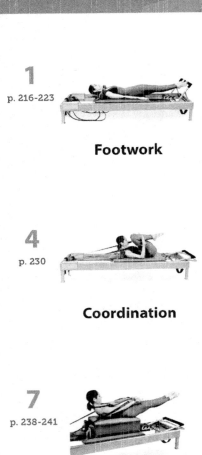

Footwork

2
p. 224

Hundred

3
p. 226-229

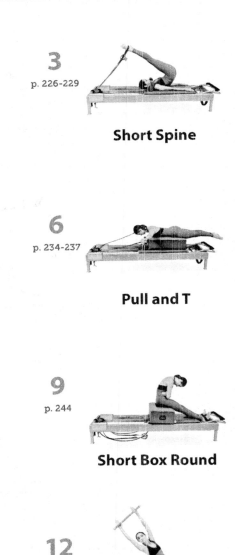

Short Spine

4
p. 230

Coordination

5
p. 232

Swan

6
p. 234-237

Pull and T

7
p. 238-241

Backstroke

8
p. 242

Teaser

9
p. 244

Short Box Round

10
p. 246

Short Box Flat

11
p. 248

Short Box Side

12
p. 250

Short Box Twist

13
p. 252

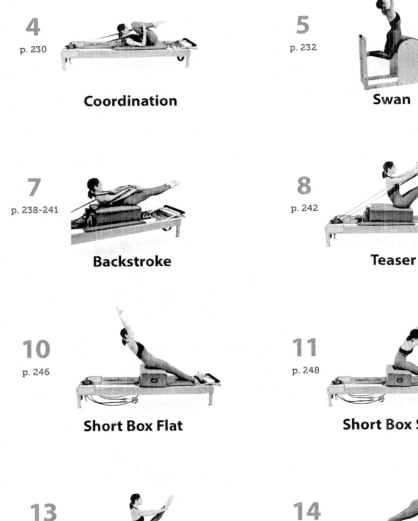

Short Box Tree

14
p. 254

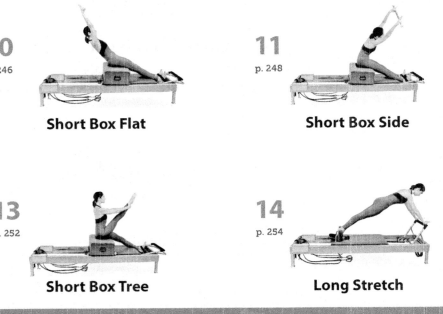

Long Stretch

15
p. 256

Down Stretch

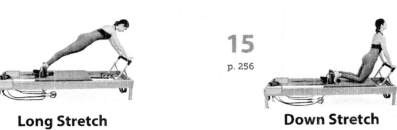

Detail

As in the matwork, the intermediate reformer exercises are integrated throughout the basic workout. There is a very specific sequence to both the basic reformer workout (p. 208-209) and the intermediate reformer workout.

16 p. 258

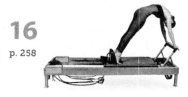

Up Stretch

17 p. 260

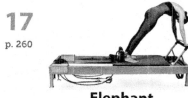

Elephant

18 p. 262

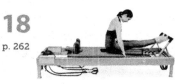

Stomach Massage Round

19 p. 264

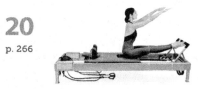

Stomach Massage Hands Back

20 p. 266

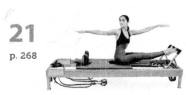

Stomach Massage Reach Up

21 p. 268

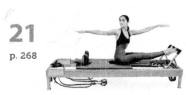

Stomach Massage Twist

22 p. 270

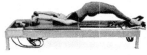

Semi-circle

23 p. 272-275

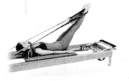

Leg Circles and Frog

24 p. 276

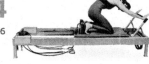

Kneeling Knee Stretches Round

25 p. 278

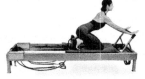

Kneeling Knee Stretches Arched

26 p. 280

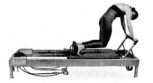

Kneeling Knee Stretches Off

27 p. 282

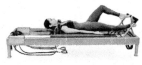

Running

28 p. 284

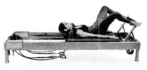

Pelvic Lift

29 p. 286

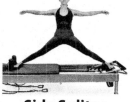

Side Splits

30 p. 288

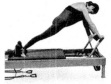

Front Splits

Reformer Parts

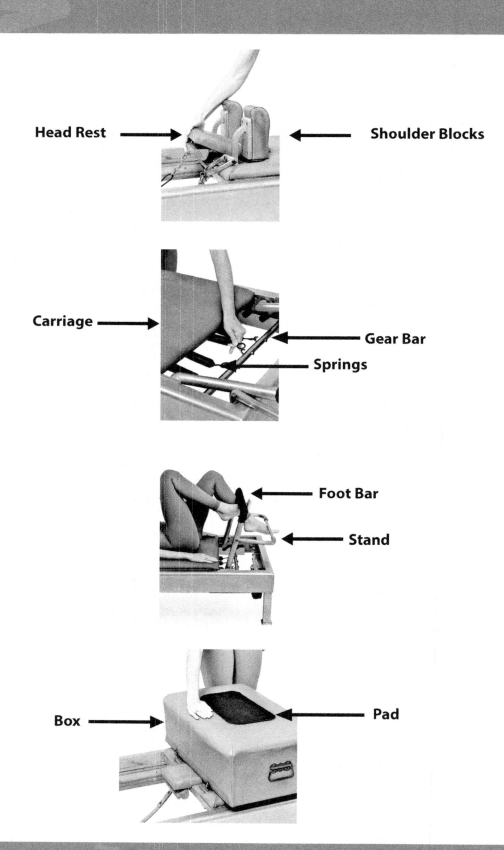

Head Rest

Shoulder Blocks

Carriage

Gear Bar

Springs

Foot Bar

Stand

Box

Pad

Detail

In addition to being familiar with your individual workout routine on the reformer, it is important to be familiar with the set-up of the Pilates apparatus. Knowing the set-up for each exercise will enhance your concentration and self-efficiency. It will also reinforce the proper techniques necessary for lifting, bending, and reaching. Before you know it, you will find yourself incorporating Pilates into every minute of your day.

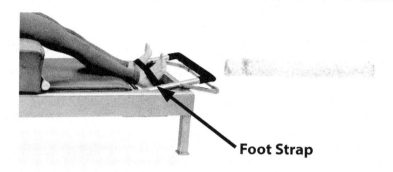

Foot Strap

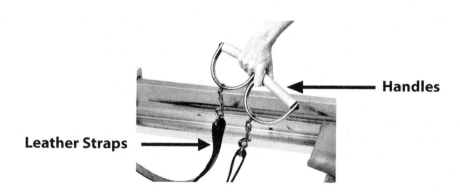

Handles

Leather Straps

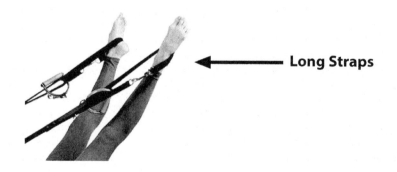

Long Straps

Well: space between the carriage and the frame.

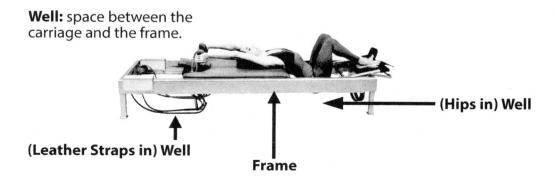

(Leather Straps in) Well

Frame

(Hips in) Well

Lying Down On The Reformer Apparatus

General Purpose:
Lying down on the reformer apparatus with a minimum of motion creates a fluid transition. It requires precision, concentration, and control.

Set-up:
2-4 springs. Foot bar and head rest are up.

Repetitions:
1 time.

Reminder:
Avoid placing your hands on the foot bar as you sit down.

My Notes:

- Pilates stance
- PH engaged
- shoulders back & down
- neck long
- open the chest

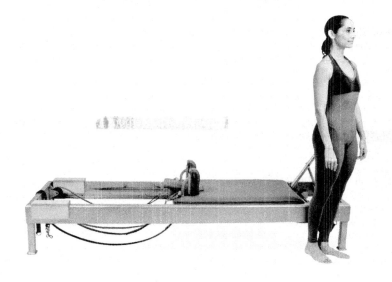

a.

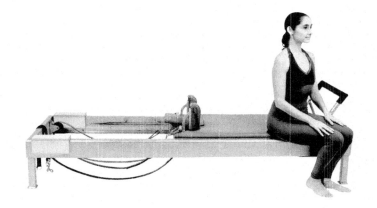

b.

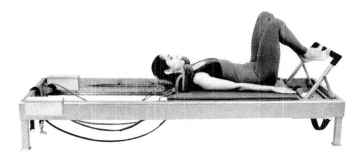

c.

Footwork Series: Toes

General Purpose:
The footwork series on the toes brings the focus to the powerhouse at the start of the workout and centers the body alignment. The pressure points on the balls of the feet correspond to the heart and lungs.

Set-up:
2-4 springs. Foot bar and head rest are up.

Repetitions:
Stretch and bend your legs 10 times.

Reminder:
Keep your knees aligned over your toes.

My Notes:

listen to the sound of the Reformer
inhale... exhale

- PH engaged
- shoulders on the mat
- arms long
- open the chest
- ribs small
- neck straight (may need 1-2 pillows)

a.

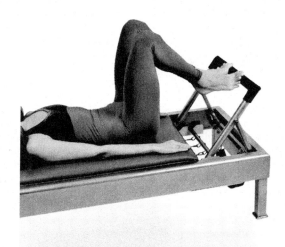

b.

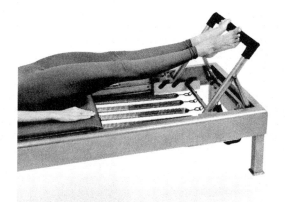

c.

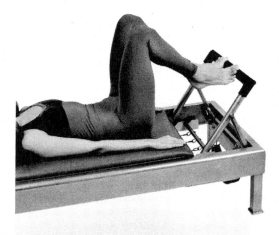

Footwork Series: Arches

General Purpose:
The footwork series on the arches brings the focus to the powerhouse at the start of the workout and centers the body alignment. The pressure points on the arches of the feet correspond to the liver and intestines.

Set-up:
2-4 springs. Foot bar and head rest are up.

Repetitions:
Stretch and bend your legs 10 times.

Reminder:
Your bottom will work more if you keep your heels curled under the bar each time you bring the carriage in.

My Notes:

- work the back of the legs
- pH engaged

a.

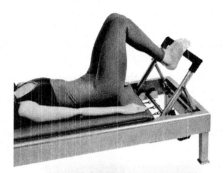

b.

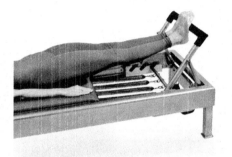

c.

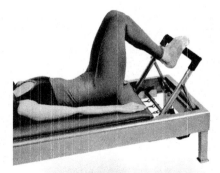

Basic / Intermediate
Footwork Series: Heels

General Purpose:
The footwork series on the heels brings the focus to the powerhouse at the start of the workout and centers the body alignment. The pressure points on the heels of the feet correspond to the kidneys and sciatic nerve.

Set-up:
2-4 springs. Foot bar and head rest are up.

Repetitions:
Stretch and bend your legs 10 times.

Reminder:
Keep your feet and ankles isolated from the movement in your legs.

My Notes:

a.

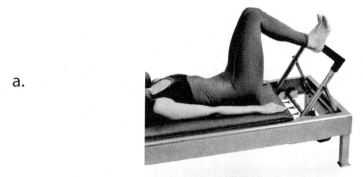

b.

c.

Footwork Series: Tendon Stretch

General Purpose:
The footwork series with the tendon stretch brings the focus to the powerhouse at the start of the workout, centers the body alignment, and stretches the back of the calves and Achilles tendons.

Set-up:
2-4 springs. Foot bar and head rest are up.

Repetitions:
Lower and lift your heels 10 times.

Reminder:
Give yourself three counts to lower your heels and three counts to lift your heels. Remember that your heels go down and up ten consecutive times <u>before</u> bringing the carriage back in.

My Notes:

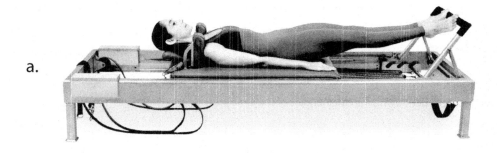

a.

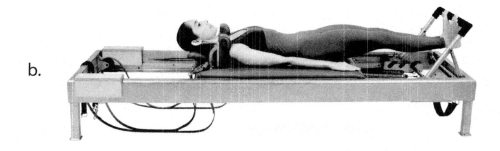

b.

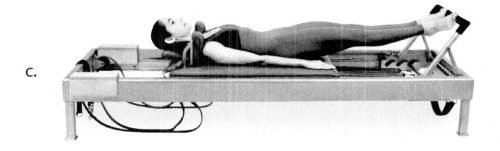

c.

Hundred

General Purpose:
The hundred warms up the body and improves endurance.

Set-up:
2-4 springs. Foot bar down. Grab the handles of the straps. Head rest can stay up.

Repetitions:
10 sets.

Reminder:
A lighter spring setting will target your powerhouse more than a heavier spring setting. A heavier spring setting will work your arms more, but will also help you hold your position in the hundred.

My Notes:

Detail

For a fluid transition from the footwork series into the hundred, use your feet to lower the foot bar.

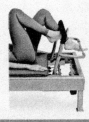

a.

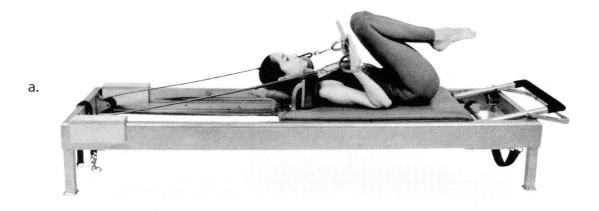

b.

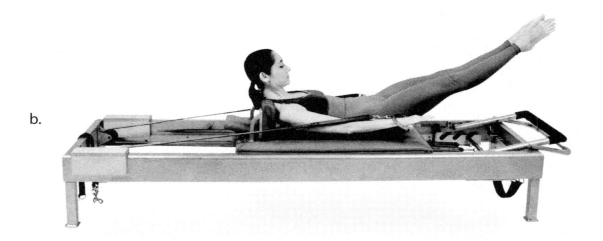

Preparing for Short Spine Massage

General Purpose:
The proper set-up for the short spine massage exercise requires powerhouse strength and uses a minimum of motion to facilitate a fluid transition.

Set-up:
2 springs. Lower the head rest and shorten the straps by threading the straps through the handles. Foot bar stays down.

Repetitions:
1 time.

Reminder:
Sit up in a teaser position to adjust the spring setting (photo A). Without moving the carriage, lift your hips to put you feet into the straps (photo D).

My Notes:

a.

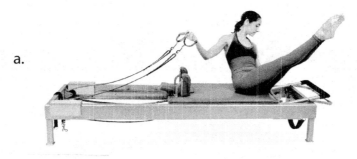

b.

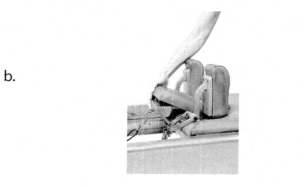

c.

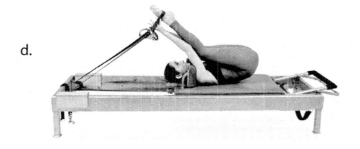

d.

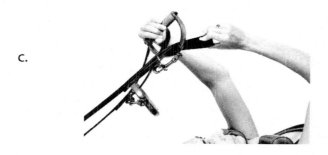

e.

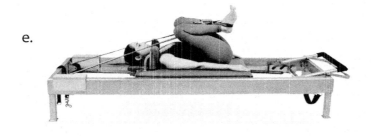

Short Spine Massage

General Purpose:
The short spine massage strengthens the powerhouse and develops articulation of the spine.

Set-up:
2 springs. Lower the head rest and shorten the straps by threading the straps through the handles. Foot bar stays down.

Repetitions:
5 times.

Reminder:
The head rest is always down for *short* spine massage (and *short* box series). Avoid using the momentum of the springs to bring your legs overhead (photo C), instead, keep your legs at working height and initiate the lift from your seat (photo B).

My Notes:

a.

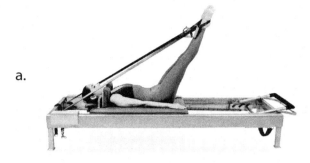

b.

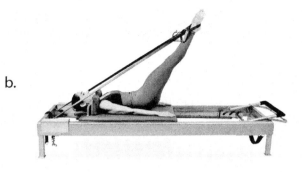

c.

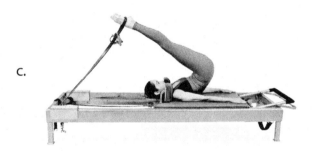

d.

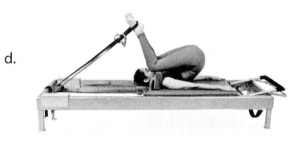

e.

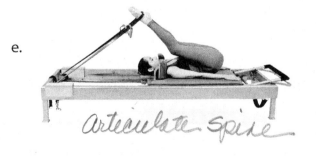

articulate spine

f.

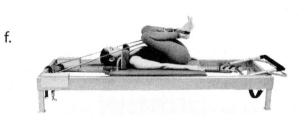

Coordination

General Purpose:
The coordination exercise improves coordination, breathing, and powerhouse strength.

Set-up:
2 springs. Head rest can go up if neck support is needed. Grab the handles. When transitioning from the short spine massage, grab both the handles and the loops of the straps, and slip the straps off your feet. Bring the carriage all the way in and pull the handles out to the end of the straps. Foot bar stays down.

Repetitions:
5 times (or 3 standard reps followed by 2 reps with the wrap around).

Reminder:
Bend your arms no more than 90 degrees in the home position to maintain tension on the straps.

My Notes:

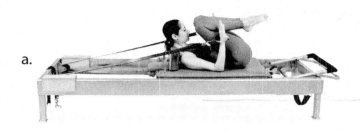

a.

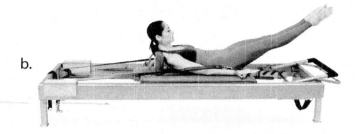

b.

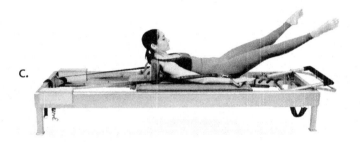

c.

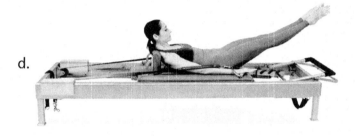

d.

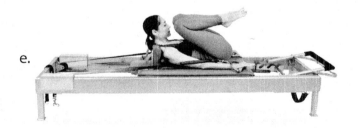

e.

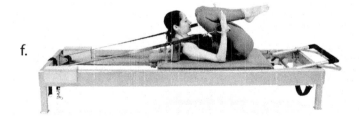

f.

Swan On The Barrel

General Purpose:
The swan on the barrel limbers the spine, opens the chest, and works the breath.

Set-up:
Drape your torso over the barrel and place your feet in Pilates stance between the bottom two ladder rungs.

Repetitions:
3 sets.

Reminder:
Set up for the long box series before heading over to the ladder barrel to perform the swan exercise. Keep the back of your neck long as you perform the back bend.

My Notes:

Horse On The Barrel

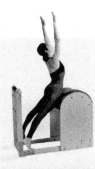

The swan exercise can also be performed with your feet on the frame of the ladder barrel.

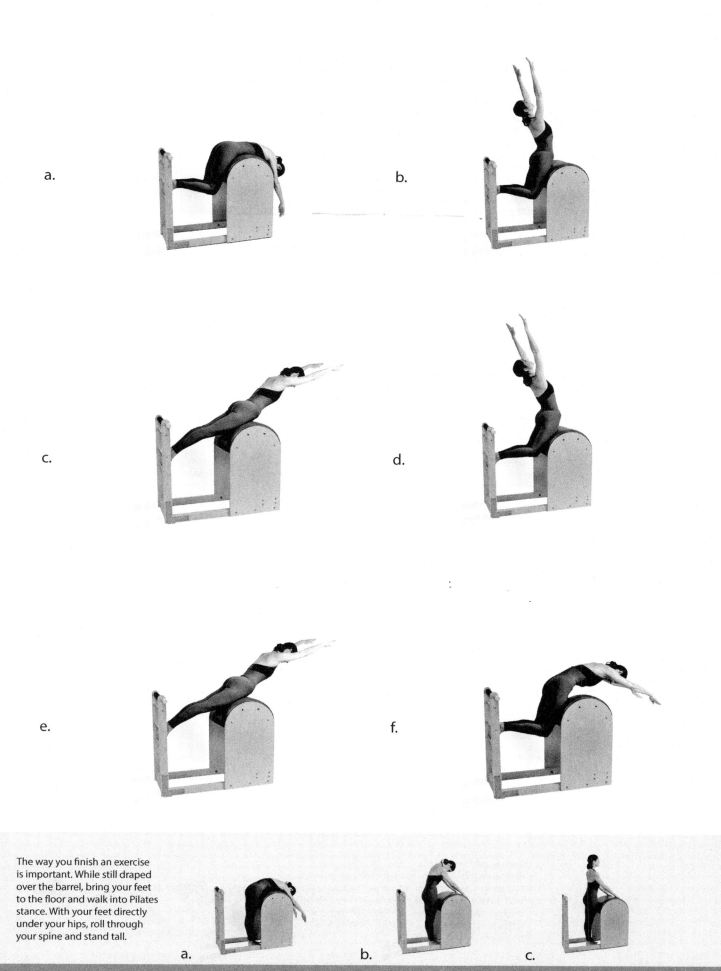

a.

b.

c.

d.

e.

f.

The way you finish an exercise is important. While still draped over the barrel, bring your feet to the floor and walk into Pilates stance. With your feet directly under your hips, roll through your spine and stand tall.

a.

b.

c.

Long Box Series: The Pull

General Purpose:
The pulling straps exercise <u>opens the chest and shoulders</u>, and <u>strengthens the upper back.</u>

Set-up:
1 spring. Place the box lengthwise on the carriage in front of the shoulder blocks. Head rest up.
Foot bar stays down.

Repetitions:
3 times.

Reminder:
As a helpful hint for remembering the spring setting, note that the first time the box goes on the carriage (long box) you use one spring to set up (the second time the box goes on the carriage for the short box series you use 2 springs). The foot bar is always down when the box is on the carriage. Your arms should remain long throughout the exercise.

My Notes:

Detail

Setting up the straps:
First lie on the box, then reach for the leather straps just above the grommets (photo A). With the leather straps in your hands, pull them towards you and grab the handles off the hooks. Keep hold of <u>both</u> the straps and the handles and let the carriage return to home position (photo B).

a. 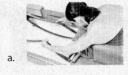   b.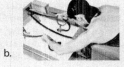

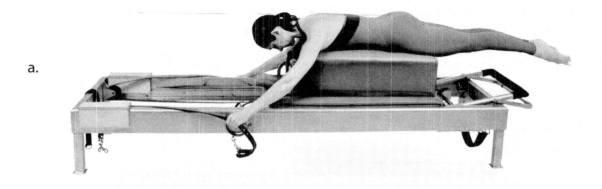

a.

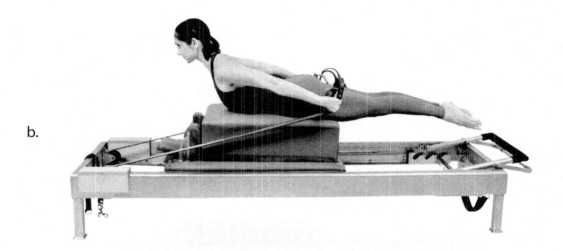

b.

Long Box Series: The "T"

General Purpose:
The "T" exercise opens the chest and shoulders and strengthens the upper back.

Set-up:
1 spring. Without letting go of the leather straps, slide the handles to the end of the straps. Keep both the strap and handle in each hand, and open your arms out to the side. Head rest stays up and foot bar stays down.

Repetitions:
3 times.

Reminder:
Your legs should hover above the foot bar at the start of the exercise and remain stationary as you lift your chest.

My Notes:

Detail

Hold the end of the straps and the handles in each hand.

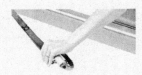

a.

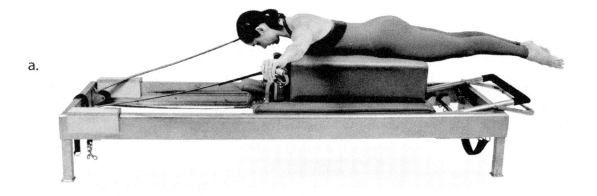

b.

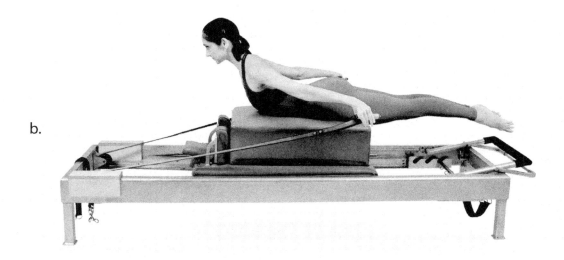

Preparing For Backstroke

General Purpose:
The proper set-up for the backstroke exercise uses a minimum of motion to facilitate a fluid transition.

Set-up:
2 springs. After performing the pull and the "T" exercises on your stomach, hold the handles side by side in one hand (photo A) to avoid crossing the straps. Step off to the side of the reformer that corresponds with the hand that is holding the handles. Use your free hand to add the second spring. Head rest stays up and foot bar stays down.

Repetitions:
1 time.

Reminder:
Place your hand (still holding one handle) on the box, your foot on the foot bar or frame of the reformer, and take a seat with your tailbone just off the edge of the box to ensure your seat will be right on the edge of the box when you lie down.

My Notes:.

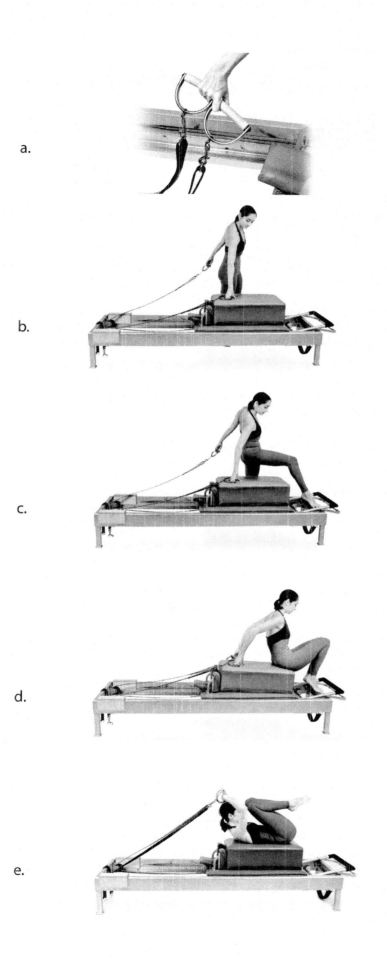

a.

b.

c.

d.

e.

Long Box Series: Backstroke

General Purpose:
The backstroke exercise deepens the powerhouse strength and improves coordination and breathing.

Set-up:
2 springs. After performing the pull and the "T" exercises on your stomach, hold the handles side by side in one hand (the dowels of the handles should not overlap). Step off to the side of the reformer that matches your hand that is holding the handles. Use your free hand to add the second spring. Head rest stays up and foot bar stays down.

Repetitions:
5 times (or 3 times forward and 2 times reverse).

Reminder:
To avoid tension in your neck, keep your gaze on your abdominals for the entire exercise, especially when your hands go up towards the sky.

My Notes:

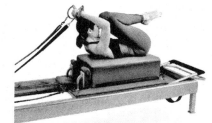

a.

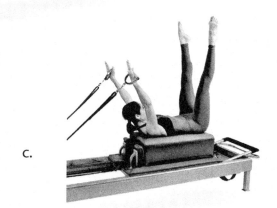

b.

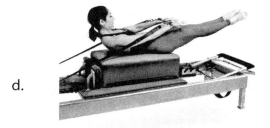

c.

d.

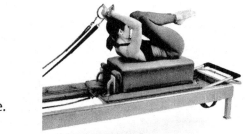

e.

Intermediate
Long Box Series:
Teaser

General Purpose:
The teaser strengthens the powerhouse, and improves the c-curve and balance control.

Set-up:
1 spring. Move back on the box a little and place the handles in one hand. Sit up with your legs in a teaser position to drop down to 1 spring. Head rest stays up and foot bar stays down.

Repetitions:
3 sets.

Reminder:
Keep the straps taut at all times.

My Notes:

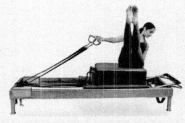

Detail

Set-up for the teaser:
Dropping one spring in preparation for the teaser is an exercise in itself.

a.

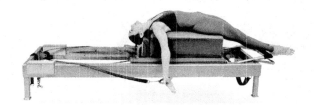

b.

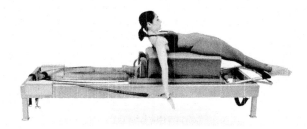

c.

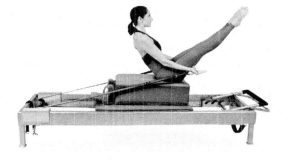

d.

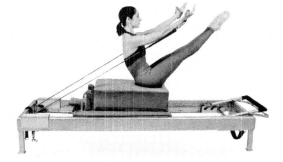

e.

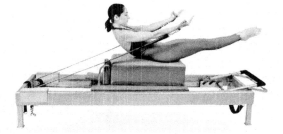

Short Box Series: Round Back

General Purpose:
The round back, also known as the hug, strengthens the powerhouse and develops the articulation of the spine.

Set-up:
2 springs. Head rest down with the box placed across the carriage and a pad placed horizontally on the box. If using a pole, place it on the carriage in front of the box. The foot bar stays down. Grab the foot straps and take a seat.

Repetitions:
3-5 times.

Reminder:
The foot bar is never in the up position when the box is on the carriage. The head rest is always down for the *short* box series (and the *short* spine massage). Squeeze your seat to avoid pressure in your back.

My Notes:

Place the box between the shoulder blocks and the hooks.

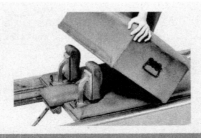

a.

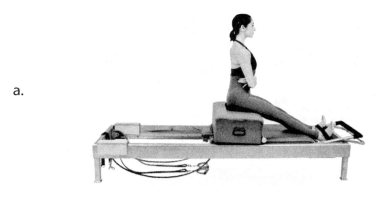

b.

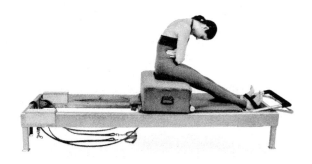

c.

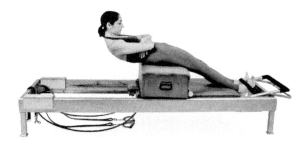

d.

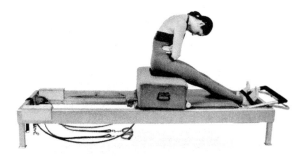

To keep tension out of your shoulders, perform the round back with your arms extended alongside your legs and your fingertips reaching towards your toes.

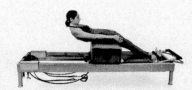

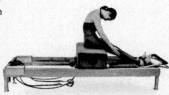

Short Box Series: Flat Back

General Purpose:
The flat back strengthens the powerhouse and lengthens the torso.

Set-up:
2 springs. Head rest and foot bar stay down with the box on the carriage.

Repetitions:
3-5 times.

Reminder:
Aim for height, not depth in this movement.

My Notes:

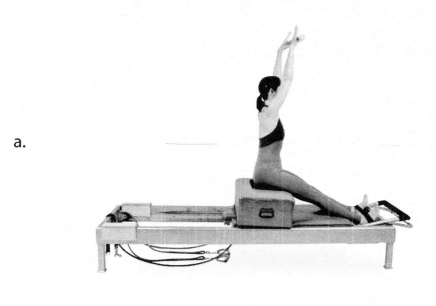

a.

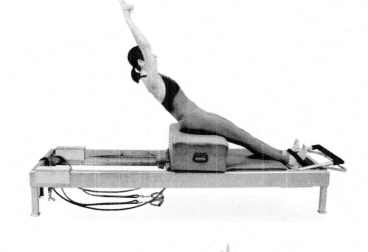

b.

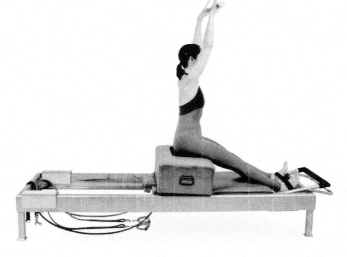

c.

Short Box Series: Side To Side

General Purpose:
The side to side lengthens the sides of the body and opens the lower back.

Set-up:
2 springs. Head rest and foot bar stay down with the box on the carriage.

Repetitions:
4 times.

Reminder:
Keep your gaze on one spot in front of you for the entire movement. *gaze high*

My Notes:

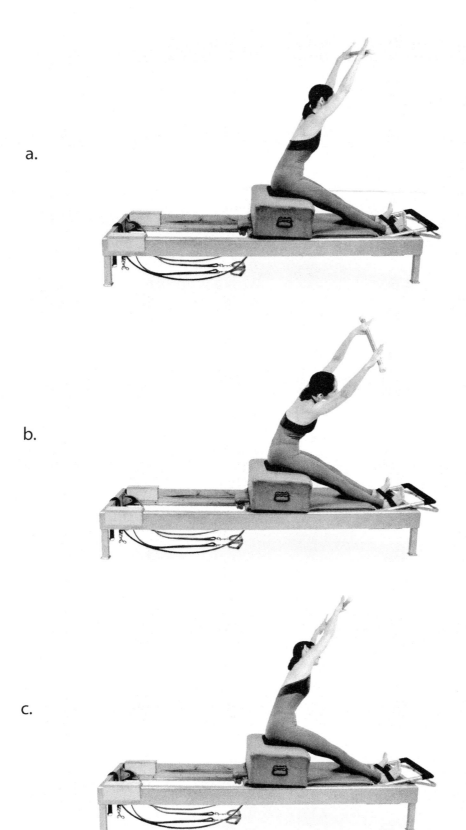

a.

b.

c.

Short Box Series: Twist

General Purpose:
The twist works the waist and strengthens the sides.

Set-up:
2 springs. Head rest and foot bar stay down with the box on the carriage.

Repetitions:
4 times.

Reminder:
Lift up and twist from your waist without moving your feet or hips.

My Notes:

a.

b.

c.

d.

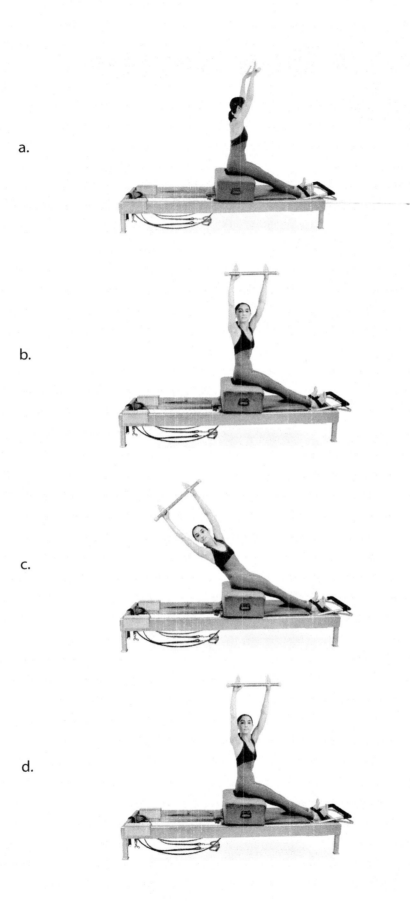

Short Box Series: Tree

General Purpose:
The tree stretches the spine, strengthens the powerhouse, and stretches the back of the leg.

Set-up:
2 springs. Head rest and foot bar stay down with the box on the carriage.

Repetitions:
Limber your leg 3 times and backbend 2 times, repeat with your other leg.

Reminder:
The focus is on stretching your spine. The stretch behind your leg is secondary.

My Notes:

Limber your leg 3 times
before the back bend.

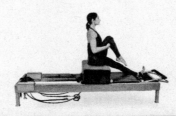
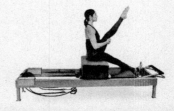

a.

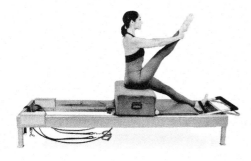

b.

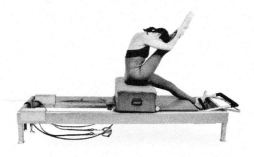

c.

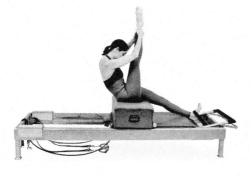

d.

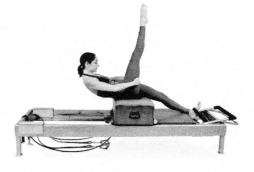

e.

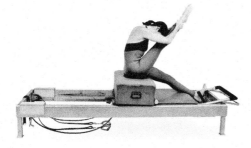

f.

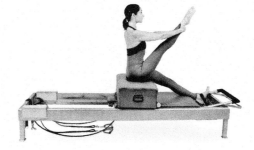

Long Stretch Series: Long Stretch

General Purpose:
The long stretch uses powerhouse strength to maintain one solid line from head to heel.

Set-up:
2 springs. The box goes to the floor, the head rest goes up with a pad, and the foot bar goes up. Place your hand on the bar before stepping up.

Repetitions:
5 times.

Reminder:
Move the carriage without letting your heels move.

My Notes:

- Shoulders over hands
- fingers together on bar

a.

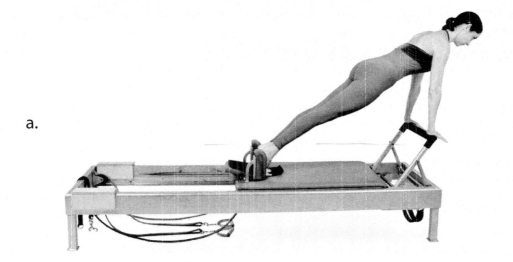

b.

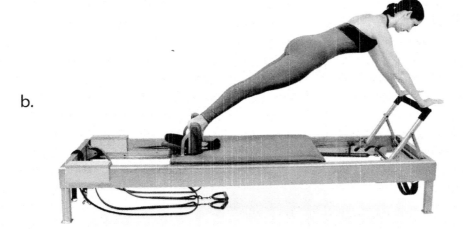

c.

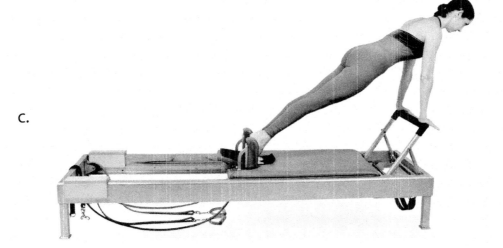

Long Stretch Series: Down Stretch

General Purpose:

The down stretch is a breathing exercise that opens the chest.

Set-up:

2 springs. Head rest and foot bar stay up.

Repetitions:

3 times.

Reminder:

Always keep your heels against the shoulder blocks. After the third repetition, hold the carriage in and place your finger tips on the bar (photo D). An easy transition from the heel of your hands to your finger tips verifies you are using your powerhouse to pull the carriage in.

My Notes:

a.

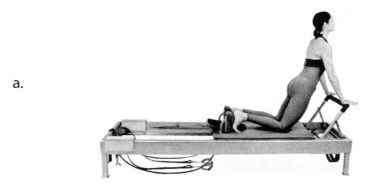

b.

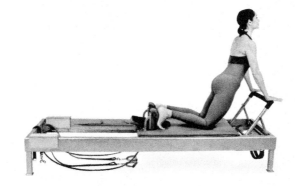

c.

d.

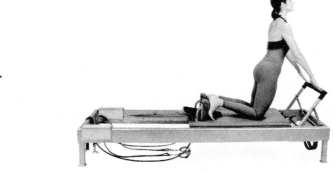

Intermediate
Long Stretch Series: Up Stretch

General Purpose:
The up stretch works the hips.

Set-up:
2 springs. Head rest and foot bar stay up.

Repetitions:
4 times.

Reminder:
Pull your stomach and ribs up towards the ceiling to bring the carriage in completely at the end of each repetition.

My Notes:.

Shoulders over hands

a.

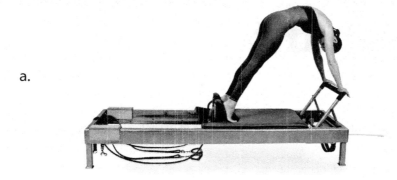

b.

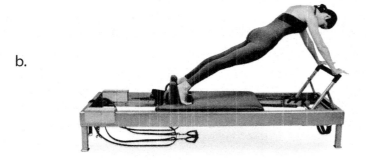

c.

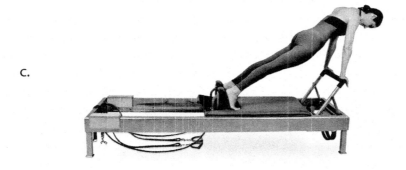

d.

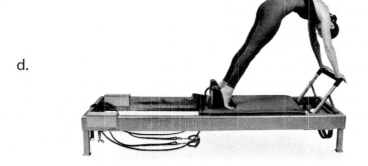

Long Stretch Series: Elephant

General Purpose:
The elephant strengthens the hips, stretches the back of the legs, and requires stabilization of the upper body.

Set-up:
2 springs. Head rest and foot bar stay up.

Repetitions:
5 times.

Reminder:
The movement of the carriage is very small in order to keep the work in your powerhouse and out of your arms and shoulders.

My Notes:

a.

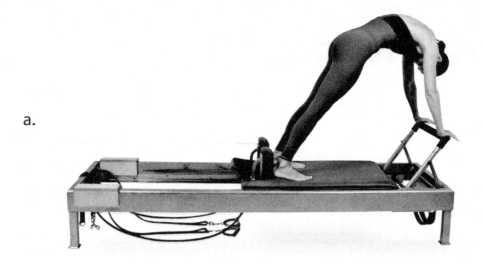

b.

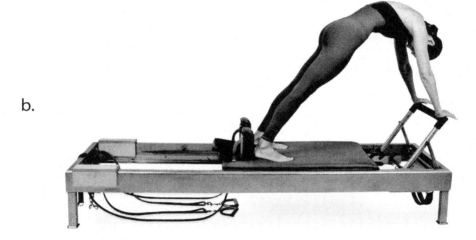

c.

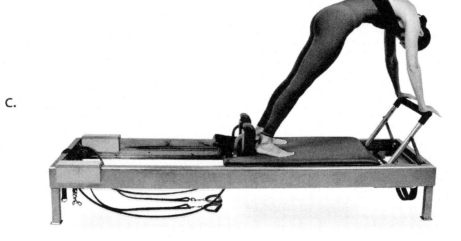

Stomach Massage Series: Round Back

General Purpose:
The stomach massage in the round back position opens the lower back, strengthens the powerhouse and the back of the arms, and stretches the legs and feet.

Set-up:
4-2 springs (ideally the same spring setting you used for the footwork series). Pad at the edge of the carriage. Head rest and foot bar stay up.

Repetitions:
10 times with tendon stretch.

Reminder:
Bring the carriage in after each tendon stretch. Even though your upper body is rounded, be sure to maintain a lift through your sides.

My Notes:

a.

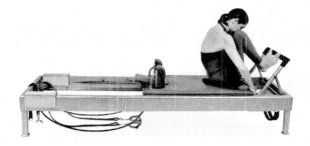

b.

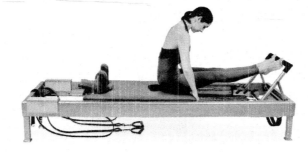

c.

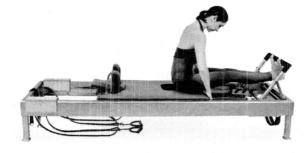

d.

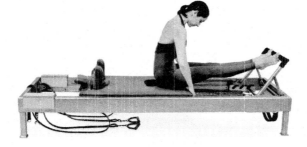

e.

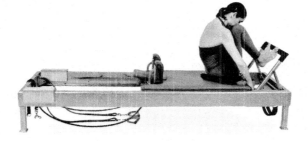

Stomach Massage Series: Hands Back

General Purpose:
The stomach massage with the hands back lengthens the lower back, opens the chest and shoulders, strengthens the powerhouse, and stretches the legs and feet.

Set-up:
3-2 springs. Head rest and foot bar stay up.

Repetitions:
10 times with tendon stretch.

Reminder:
Try to keep your chest lifted as the carriage comes in.

My Notes:

a.

b.

c.

d.

e.

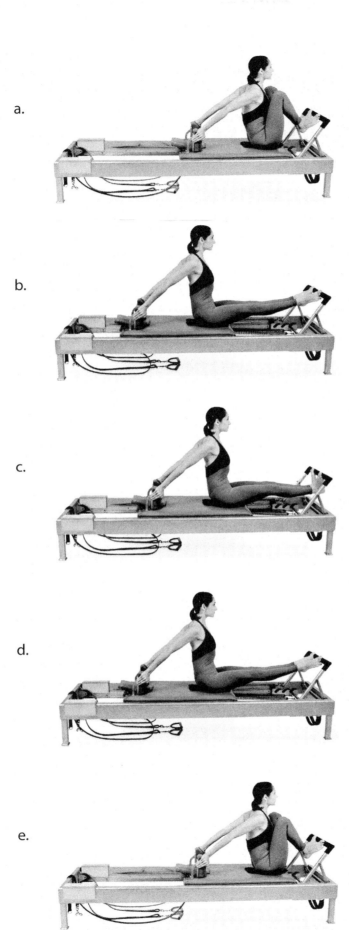

Stomach Massage Series: Reach Up

General Purpose:
The stomach massage with the reach up lifts the powerhouse.

Set-up:
2 springs. Head rest and foot bar stay up.

Repetitions:
4 times.

Reminder:
Try to keep your shoulders aligned over your hips throughout the exercise.

My Notes:

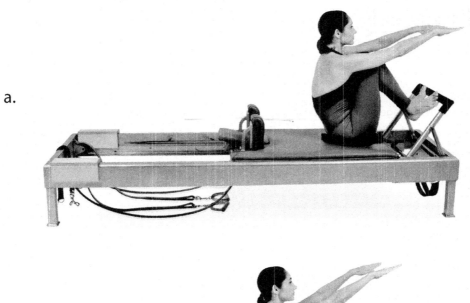

a.

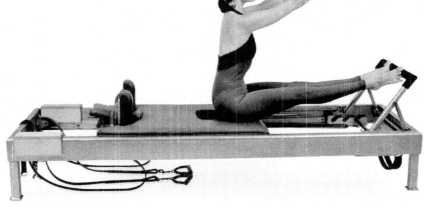

b.

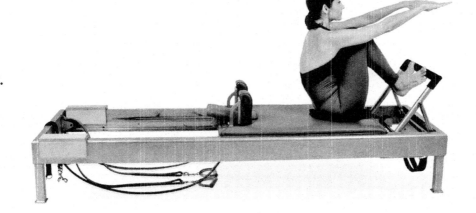

c.

Stomach Massage Series: Twist

General Purpose:
The stomach massage with the twist works the waist and opens the sides.

Set-up:
2 springs. Head rest and foot bar stay up.

Repetitions:
6 times.

Reminder:
Keep your heels together and lifted throughout the exercise.

My Notes:

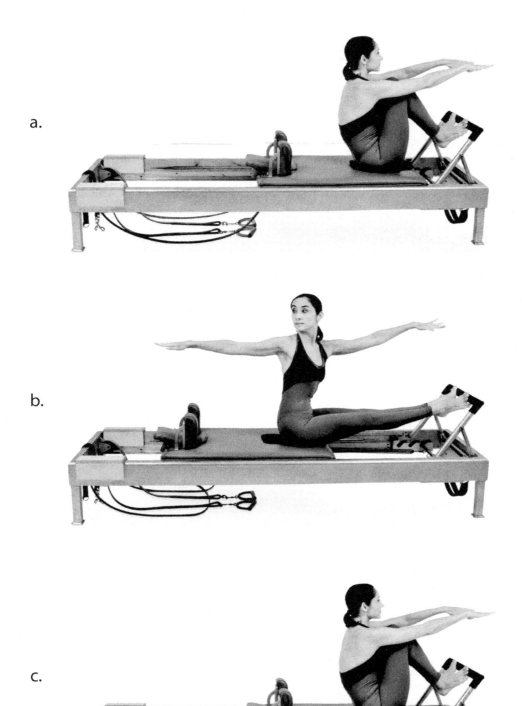

a.

b.

c.

Semi-Circle

General Purpose:
The semi-circle develops the articulation of the spine, opens the chest, increases control in the hips, and stretches the thighs.

Set-up:
2 springs. Lower the foot bar, and cover the foot bar and frame with two pads placed side by side. Head rest stays up.

Repetitions:
3 times and reverse.

Reminder:
Set up the long straps for the leg circle series and place them on the hooks behind the shoulder blocks prior to lying down for the semi-circle. To begin the semi-circle, roll through your spine as you lower your back into the well. Squeeze your seat to keep your hips even.

My Notes:

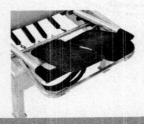

Pad placement for the semi-circle.

a.

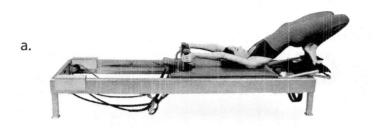

b.

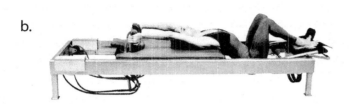

c.

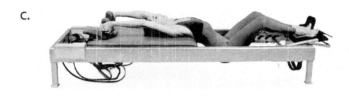

d.

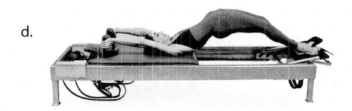

e.

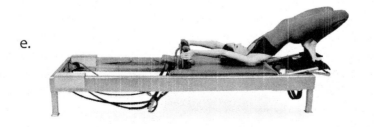

Leg Circles

General Purpose:
The leg circles work the legs evenly with control.

Set-up:
2 springs. To extend the straps for leg circles, thread the long straps through the handle and the loop of each leather strap. Head rest stays up. Foot bar stays down.

Repetitions:
5 times and reverse.

Reminder:
If you performed the semi-circle exercise, the long straps should have been set up for these leg circles prior to lying down for the semi-circle. While performing the leg circles, watch your feet for symmetry as you circle your legs.

My Notes:

Thread the long straps through the handle and the loop of each leather strap.

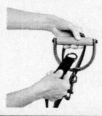

a.

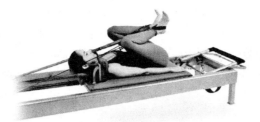

b.

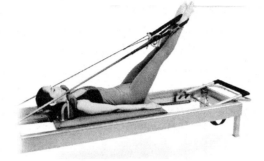

c.

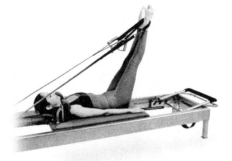

d.

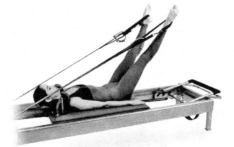

e.

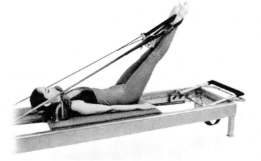

Frog

General Purpose:
The frog exercise tones the legs and develops control.

Set-up:
2 springs. Head rest stays up. Foot bar stays down. Long straps as used in the leg circle exercise.

Repetitions:
6 times.

Reminder:
When extending your legs, be sure the leather straps hover just above, but do not touch the shoulder blocks.

My Notes:

a.

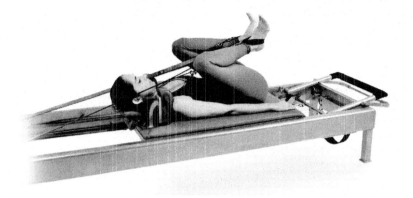

b.

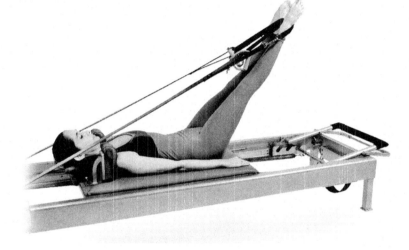

c.

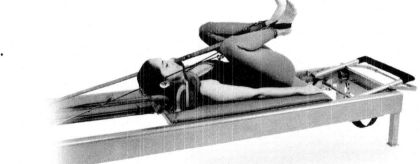

Kneeling Knee Stretch Series: Round

General Purpose:
The kneeling knee stretch series in the round back position opens the lower back, strengthens the seat, and requires stabilization of the upper body as the legs move.

Set-up:
2 springs. Foot bar up. Head rest stays up.

Repetitions:
6-8 times.

Reminder:
To work your bottom, keep your hips down near your heels at the start and try not to lift your hips as you push the carriage out.

My Notes:

a.

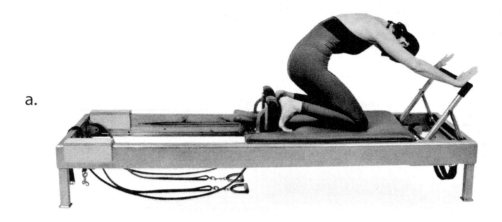

b.

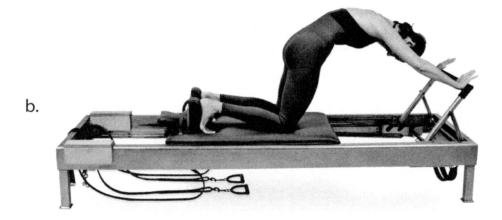

c.

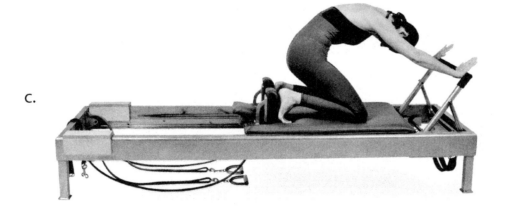

Kneeling Knee Stretch Series: Arched

General Purpose:
The kneeling knee stretch series in the arched back position opens the chest, strengthens the seat, and requires stabilization of the upper body as the legs move.

Set-up:
2 springs. Head rest and foot bar stay up.

Repetitions:
6-8 times.

Reminder:
Keep the back of your neck long and your stomach pulled in.

My Notes:

a.

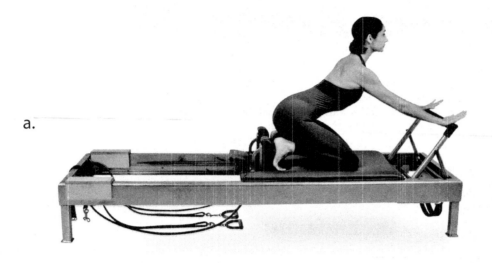

b.

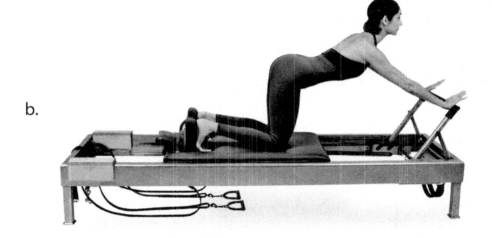

c.

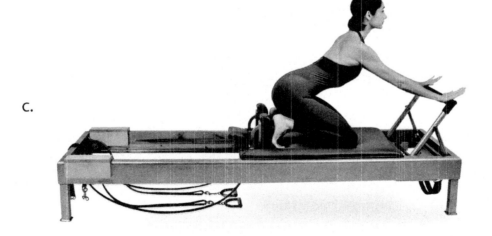

Kneeling Knee Stretch Series: Knees Off

General Purpose:
The kneeling knee stretch series with the knees off the carriage strengthens the legs and stomach, and requires stabilization of the upper body as the legs move.

Set-up:
2 springs. Head rest and foot bar stay up.

Repetitions:
10-20 times.

Reminder:
Keep the heels of your feet glued to the shoulder blocks and your shoulders over the gear bar throughout the exercise. A box can be used to shorten the carriage if your proportions warrant it.

My Notes:

a.

b.

c.

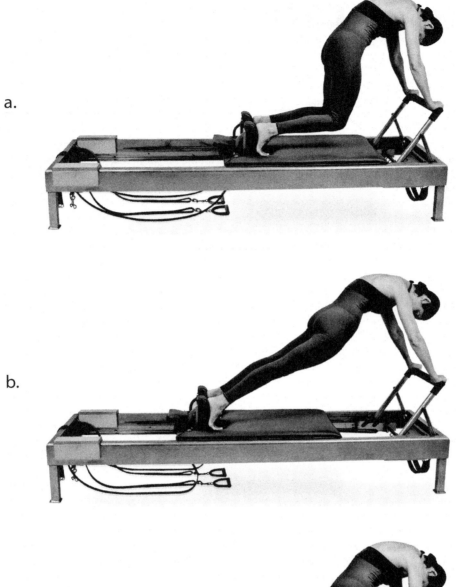

Running

General Purpose:
The running exercise is a cool down exercise. It brings the workout full circle by returning to the lying down position used at the start of the workout.

Set-up:
4-2 springs (ideally the same spring setting you used for the footwork series). Head rest and foot bar stay up.

Repetitions:
20 times.

Reminder:
Both heels are lifted to start and finish the running exercise. The accent is on the upbeat during the prancing movement.

My Notes:

a.
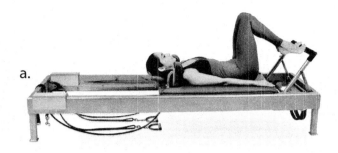

b.
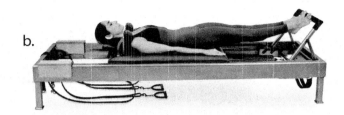

c.
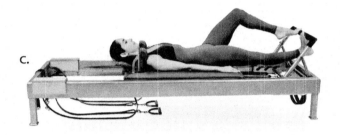

d.
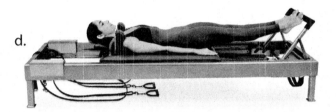

e.
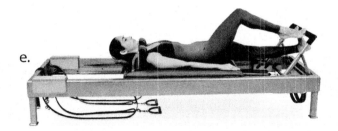

f.
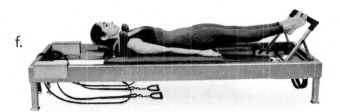

Pelvic Lift

General Purpose:
The pelvic lift strengthens the back of the legs and bottom.

Set-up:
1-4 springs. Head rest and foot bar stay up. Place your arches on the corners of the foot bar with your legs and feet turned out, and your knees over your toes.

Repetitions:
10 times.

Reminder:
Keep your waist on the carriage as you lift your hips. Basic level: lift your hips about four fingers high off the carriage. Intermediate level: lift your hips only two fingers high off the carriage. Lower your hips onto the mat after bringing the carriage in only on the last repetition.

My Notes:

a.

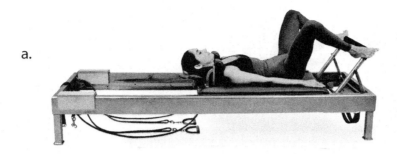

b.

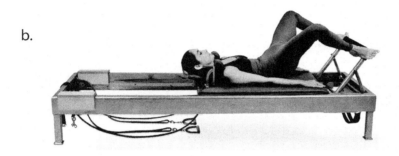

c.

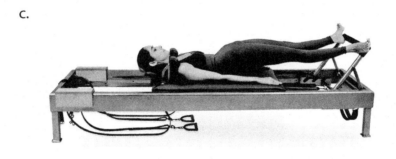

d.

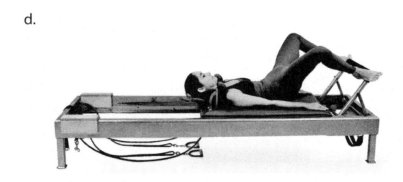

Intermediate

Side Splits

General Purpose:
The side splits work the body from the inside out, strengthen the inner and outer thighs, and improve posture.

Set-up:
1-2 springs. Foot bar goes down. Head rest stays up. Place one pad on the carriage in the crease of the shoulder block closest to you. Place a second pad on the frame of the reformer (under the foot bar), directly across from the pad on the carriage.

Repetitions:
3 sets on each side. There is a 3 count hold each time the carriage goes out and each time it comes in.

Reminder:
To start, step up on the carriage, then place one foot on the pad on the frame before your other foot wiggles out towards the pad in front of the shoulder block. Lift your powerhouse (not your shoulders) to bring the carriage in.

My Notes:

Detail

Pad placement for the side splits.

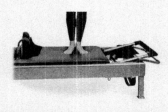